Getting to Dry

Getting to Dry

How to Help Your Child Overcome Bedwetting

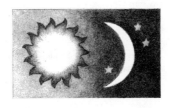

Max Maizels, M.D.
Diane Rosenbaum, Ph.D.
Barbara Keating, R.N., M.S.

with editorial assistance from
Reno Lovison

The Harvard Common Press
Boston, Massachusetts

All matters regarding your health or your children's health require medical supervision. The authors and publishers disclaim any liability arising, whether directly or indirectly, from the use of this book.

The Harvard Common Press
535 Albany Street
Boston, Massachusetts 02118

Printed in the United States of America
Printed on acid-free paper

Library of Congress Cataloging-in-Publication Data

Maizels, Max.
     Getting to dry : how to help your child overcome bedwetting / Max Maizels, Diane Rosenbaum, Barbara Keating.
        p. cm.
     Includes index.
     ISBN 1-55832-130-6 (hardcover : alk. paper).—
ISBN 1-55832-131-4 (pbk. : alk. paper)
     1. Enuresis—Popular works.   I. Rosenbaum, Diane.
II. Keating, Barbara.   III. Title.
  RJ476.E6M34   1999
  618.92'849—dc21   97-36913
                              CIP

Special bulk-order discounts are available on this and other Harvard Common Press books. Companies and organizations may purchase books for premiums or for resale, or may arrange a custom edition, by contacting the Marketing Director at the address above.

Cover design by Kathleen Herlihy-Paoli, Inkstone Design
Text design by Joyce C. Weston
Illustrations by Susan Aldridge
10 9 8 7 6 5 4

This book is dedicated to all the children who have suffered humiliation, shame, or even punishment because they wet, by day or by night, and to all the children who are trying to overcome their wetting problem and get to dry.

The authors are deeply grateful for the help
and support of their families over the years:
Evelyn and Michael W. Maizels,
Joel and Julia Resnick, and Bill, Katie,
and Nicole Keating.

Contents

Preface

By Max Maizels, M.D.

THIS BOOK is a guide for parents and children who are trying to cope with and overcome nighttime wetting, daytime wetting, or both. Drawn from the experience of our team of wetting specialists who have helped hundreds of families with similar problems, the methods and practical advice offered here are designed to put the control largely in your hands. We will show you first how to understand and then how to resolve your child's wetting condition. Along the way, you will need to consult a health professional, but you will help direct the treatment: you will determine the likely causes of your child's wetting, and you will develop a strategy for solving the problem and helping your child learn to stop wetting. In the end, you, and your child who wets, will master the attitude and techniques that will ensure long-term success.

In order for your child to begin making progress toward complete dryness, you—and any others involved in the care of your child—need to understand that overcoming wetness can be a major undertaking. There are no simple solutions. Our approach requires a relatively small contribution of your time before you see results. However, considering how much time and effort you probably now spend dealing with the problem, we think the investment is worth it. Our experience has clearly shown that the children and families who are most committed to changing their situation are the ones who most often succeed in doing so.

Other adults who interact with children will also find our approach useful. We believe our program will be especially helpful to:

- schoolteachers and day-care providers
- mental health professionals
- health-care professionals, especially pediatricians, pediatric nurses, and school nurses
- counselors at overnight or day camps
- leaders of youth activities for girls or boys
- coaches, especially in leagues that involve travel
- grandparents
- teens who babysit

To all those who care for children, we have a simple request. Respect the dignity of those who wet; they do so not because they choose to be wet, but because they haven't yet learned how to be dry. This book can help you teach them.

The Try for Dry Program

In August 1983, crowded inside a sweltering Chicago apartment, a small group of newly trained Children's Memorial Hospital doctors—including Dr. Diane Rosenbaum, Dr. Mark Stein (now at the Children's National Medical Center in Washington, D.C.), and myself—and our spouses sat eating pizza. I had just finished four years of surgical training at Northwestern University's Department of Urology and eagerly awaited the surgical challenges of reconstructing the all-too-common birth defects of children. I explained to the others that one major, unexpected problem nagged at me, one for which most doctors, including myself, are not prepared: how to help children who wet at night.

Diane revealed similar difficulties with her patients: "If only I could be sure that the children didn't have urological birth defects, I bet I could get them dry." I replied: "If only *I* could be sure that the children didn't have important psychopathology, I bet *I* could get them dry." The spark of an idea seemed to crackle in the room: We should work together, urologist and psychologist, to pool our expertise and bring to bear on the problem a comprehensive treatment program.

In the 1980s, such collaboration on wetting problems was unknown. Physicians simply had not organized their resources into a recognized, proven method to evaluate, diagnose, and treat the condition. Medical students and residents received no formal training in wetting disorders. Practitioners recognized that some unknown number of children wet because of birth defects of their urinary tract (a malpositioned ureter, say, or a blocked bladder), so they at least could try to rule out this problem in their patients by referring them to a pediatric urologist. Every now and then, in turn, a pediatric urologist would find a birth defect and correct it surgically, enabling the child to become dry. This very good experience led physicians to refer more and more children who bedwet to urologists. However, the majority of those children simply did not need surgery. So pediatric urologists were "stuck" with boatloads of wet children for whom surgery was not the answer—but we had no clear course to follow. Parents were equally at a loss for ways to help their wet children.

At first I tried the treatments I had seen others use—and hoped for the best. But such traditional methods were inconsistent and unpredictable. Sometimes moisture alarms attached to the child's underwear worked, but sometimes not. Sometimes medications worked, but they also commonly caused problematic weight loss, sleeplessness, and hair loss. Also, I wanted to be certain that I was not overlooking important psychological issues in the lives of the children and their families.

So, after nurse and parent educator Barbara Keating, R.N., M.S., came on board, we three authors set out as a team to evaluate and treat children with wetting problems.

It took about five years to develop and refine our approach, which targets four causes of wetting:

Problem	Solution
Deep sleep	When asleep, the child wears a moisture alarm that sounds at the first drops of urine.
Small bladder capacity	The child takes a medication that lessens the feeling of urgency to urinate.
Irregular bowel movements	The child follows a toileting regimen to encourage daily bowel movements.
Food sensitivities	By following an elimination diet, the child tries to isolate foods that may hinder bladder control.

In 1986, we decided to focus our efforts through a new program, the Center to Assist Physicians in the Regulation of Enuresis (CARE). During our five years working as CARE, we saw lots of children, and our confidence and proficiency in our process grew. In 1992, we realized that in order to significantly transform the treatment of bedwetting, we needed not only to treat children and advise their pediatricians, but also to educate other health professionals and lay people. With this objective in mind, we initiated the Program in Pediatric Enurology and the Try for Dry program at Chicago's Children's Memorial Hospital. The Program in Pediatric Enurology provides postgraduate training for community-based health-care professionals in the diagnosis and treatment of wetting problems in children. The Try for Dry program, upon which this book is based, offers enuresis materials and treatment to children and their families. We often help families and their own doctors devise the best methods to work together to remedy the wetting.

The Try for Dry program meets a long-standing need for a recognized, focused attack on childhood wetting problems. On the Internet and in magazines, you will find plenty of companies and nonprofit organizations offering a variety of solutions to wetting, as well as products ranging from custom-made absorbent underwear to holistic tablets. Some of the information provided is very good, but most other approaches to the problem tend to be somewhat passive and slow-moving. They may succeed in the long run, but we believe there is a better way. The Try for Dry program presented in this book is the first aggressive, carefully organized and implemented assault on wetting problems, especially bedwetting.

IN OUR COUNTRY today, millions of desperate parents and their children struggle with routine toilet training. When a child fails to achieve dryness "normally," the parents yearn for answers: "What should we do next?" Beyond the brief tips in encyclopedic parenting manuals and the specialized (and often costly) programs built around a single "guaranteed" technique or device, there are very few accessible, comprehensive resources out there.

With this book, we hope to answer that call for help. Arranged in three parts—"Understanding the Problem," "Finding the Solutions," and "Following Through"—*Getting to Dry* will steer you and your child toward permanent dryness. You (and your family, in consultation with your health-care provider) will drive the process: you and your child will gather the information, choose and implement the components of the treatment plan, and work past any trouble spots along the way.

Helping a child to master his or her bodily functions can be tremendously challenging. No matter what methods they try, children who wet and their families must have a firm commitment to use any chosen treatment *consistently* in order to resolve a wetting problem. The families we have helped have told us over and over that, compared with the time and effort they used to spend struggling with the mess and stress of bedwetting, the treatment plan came as a welcome relief. Using the proven techniques adapted here, you will spend your time wisely, engaged in positive rather than negative efforts. That is, you will spend more time building successful behaviors and less time reacting to wetting incidents. By investing your time in learning the likely causes of your child's wetting and focusing on solutions that work best for him, you will significantly increase your child's chances of reaching dryness.

Using This Book

We know that parents are pressed for time, even more so today than in the recent past, so we have structured the book to accommodate the needs of a variety of readers. *If you are just beginning to confront your child's bedwetting problem, we suggest that you read each chapter in sequence.* Part One explains the various possible causes of wetting and provides an overall understanding of the problem. Part Two reviews how treatments may be structured. Part Three details the typical courses of action for following through with treatments that are successful and explains what to do when they are not.

- Chapter 1 describes the various forms of wetting, gives advice on simplifying clean-up, and lays out a plan of action.
- Chapter 2 is devoted to the physiological factors that likely cause wetting.

- Chapter 3 examines some common misconceptions about children who wet, the possible psychological contributors to wetting, and the effects the problem may have on your child's self-image.

- Chapter 4 leads you through the information-gathering stage of the program: completing our brief questionnaire, keeping an observation diary, and visiting your health-care provider.

- Chapter 5 matches the causes that you've identified with the best-odds solutions. Here is where you will also find a comprehensive discussion of the primary tool for curing wetting, the enuresis alarm.

- Chapter 6 presents the additional tools designed to treat the specific causes of your child's wetting. When used in combination with the enuresis alarm, these treatments are highly successful.

- Chapter 7 offers incentives and other motivators that you may adapt in order to help your child stay on the path toward dryness.

- Chapter 8 contains detailed instructions about gradually completing the program once your child has achieved dryness—and what to do if wetting returns.

- Chapter 9 is a problem-solving resource, a collection of common solutions to the complications—practical and philosophical—you may encounter along the way.

If you and your family have been struggling with and slowly learning more and more about bedwetting for some time, you may want to begin with Chapter 4, so that you can start collecting the information you will need to develop your child's dryness program in Chapters 5 and 6. However, we encourage even the most experienced veterans of wetness to review the common causes and effects of bedwetting, as we describe them in Chapters 1 through 3. You may learn something new or perhaps remember details you had forgotten. Also, even if you choose to skip reading the introductory chapters, you may want to share them with close relatives or friends who have regular contact with the child who wets. If you decide to enlist their help with the dryness program, they will need to understand the rationale behind the individual dryness treatments.

In the back of the book, you will find a number of resources, including a glossary of frequently used words, a brief summary of the most common disorders of incontinence, and a directory of organizations and product suppliers.

AFTER WETTING and its attendant difficulties have faded from your daily life, we hope that you and your child will continue to benefit from the experiences you share during this time. In hundreds of children we have helped, we have witnessed an enhanced sense of self-control and self-esteem, once they have achieved permanent dryness. In addition, the children and their families have shown the satisfaction that comes with tackling a persistent problem and beating it, together. On behalf of our entire Try for Dry team, I wish you the same success.

Max Maizels, M.D.
Division of Urology
Children's Memorial Hospital
Chicago, Illinois

NOTE: For more information about the services and materials available from the Try for Dry program, or to contact the authors via E-mail, visit our Website at this address:

http://www.tryfordry.com

Introduction

WETTING PROBLEMS, whether nighttime or daytime, are unacceptable topics for discussion in almost any gathering—often even among family members. Most people feel uncomfortable talking—and hearing—about bodily functions, and many incorrectly assume that children who wet must be troubled behaviorally or emotionally. Precisely because talking about wetting is taboo, children who wet and those who love them tend to suffer silently—for a while, anyway.

Desperately Seeking Help

SUBJECT: BED SOAKING!

Does anyone out there have my son's problem with bedwetting? He is almost seven years old. He has been daytime trained since he was three. He has to wear a diaper to bed. If we are not careful watching his fluid intake, he will soak through his diaper at night. Sometimes we are careful and he still soaks through. We started buying those new [brand-name undergarments] because they said they were more absorbent, but after a couple of weeks we found them to be no better. I have asked our pediatrician about it; he just says he should grow out of it. He looks as if he's a long ways from that. What'll I do in the meantime?

This message was posted on an Internet electronic bulletin board. Millions of parents each year in the United States agonize over their children's wetting problems in just the same way:

> *"Am I doing the right things?"*
> *"Should I make her wear diapers?"*
> *"We've tried prohibiting drinking after 7:00 P.M., having him get up to pee at 3:00 A.M., and even insisting that he do his own laundry, but nothing works."*
> *"Maybe my mother's right. Maybe he has a psychological problem."*
> *"My doctor said to just wait until my daughter is seven. But I want to fix this now!"*

Acting on the advice of friends or well-meaning relatives, parents may decide to offer their child an extravagant reward for staying dry (such as a new bicycle). Or they may fall back on timeworn emotional manipulation: shame ("You're just too lazy to get up!") or blame ("All the boys on your father's side did it. It's really your father's fault!"). Most parents can maintain their composure, but when they are exhausted and angry, some may force a wet, groggy child to change his pajamas and sheets—and then to go sleep in the bathtub! Some parents have even injured their child emotionally or physically, or both, through excessive punishment. You may have felt some degree of the same desperation and the overwhelming need for good advice, only to have found very little.

Because wetting conditions are still viewed today fundamentally as psychological problems, occurring mainly in children whose families have *psychosocial* problems, there is little organized *medical* treatment available for them. For example, in the diagnostic manual for the psychiatric profession, *Diagnostic and Statistical Manual–IV,* enuresis appears as a psychiatric diagnosis.

Although such a diagnosis may be applicable to individuals with a psychiatric disorder, enuresis is in fact also listed as a medical condition in the *International Classification of Diseases*. Many doctors refrain from active treatment of routine bedwetting until the child is seven years old. After making sure that the child's physical examination, urine analysis, and urine stream are normal, the doctor will typically advise parents to just wait a little longer, in the hope that the child will outgrow it.

In fact, daytime and nighttime wetting are primarily physiological problems, and they are potentially as responsive to treatment as many other medical conditions. Why should so many children and families wait for years to outgrow the problem? Don't children have a right to be dry?

We think they do. This book deals with overcoming wetting when you and your child have decided not to wait months or years hoping the problem will magically disappear.

The Medical View of Wetting

Throughout history people have consistently labeled children who wet as shameful, bad, or lazy (or all three). This "blaming the victim" helps explain why wetting has not yet achieved the legitimacy generally given to other medical symptoms, such as wheezing due to asthma, epileptic seizures, and so on. As the medical community has come to understand how allergens cause wheezing, people have stopped saying, "Oh! He is just a sickly child." When children have "fits" due to epilepsy, people no longer blame the child for acting out. These problems now have recognized medical evaluation and treatment plans. The burden of guilt is now where it belongs: on the causes of the symptoms, whether the environment, disease, or some physiological problem.

IS WETTING A SYMPTOM, A PROBLEM, OR BOTH?

The procedure is not quite so straightforward for wetting. Perhaps doctors and other health-care professionals have not yet perfected the medical management of wetting because we have differing assumptions. Is wetting a symptom or a problem? If it is considered to be only a symptom, then why treat it? If, on the other hand, wetting is seen as a problem resulting from at least four possible causes:

1. failure of sleep arousal,
2. small bladder size,
3. neurological problems, and
4. overproduction of urine . . .

then we should treat it!

Perhaps the child wets at night because he feels tremendous anxieties during the day. Or conversely, perhaps the child is anxious all day because he is fearful of wetting the bed at night. As a first step in diagnosing the root problem, parents and doctor must agree on an approach: Are they dealing with a symptom caused by a medical problem, a problem behavior with an unknown cause, or both?

A doctor's job, in a nutshell, is to look for the underlying cause of the symptoms that she sees. When you visit a doctor because you are concerned about, say, a rash on your ankles, the doctor does her medical detective work (takes a history, does a physical examination, perhaps orders a test) and tries to solve the mystery for you. She may determine that you have a rash because you're allergic to the elastic in your socks.

Doctors generally don't take the simple symptom of wetting as seriously as, say, shortness of breath. Why? Probably because we recognize that shortness of breath itself is very distressing, and that it usually signals a serious underlying medical problem, such as asthma or heart disease. Also, the medical community knows how to treat the causes of shortness of breath. We take the symptom seriously because it can have life-threatening results and because we are confident in our ability to find and treat the problem.

Unfortunately, such is not the case with wetting. On the surface, doctors might ask what problems the symptoms cause. "Just wet clothes and sheets? Disrupted sleep?" The fact that wetting can result in such difficulties as poor self-esteem, social isolation, family conflict, and desperation does not usually stimulate an aggressive medical treatment.

Our team keeps the horse in front of the cart. We feel that parents, not just doctors, should judge the negative effects their child is experiencing due to wetting. Doctors should focus on figuring out if the symptom of wetting arises from a medical problem. In our approach, the medical staff follows the family's lead:

1. The family decides that their child's bedwetting is causing enough distress to warrant action.
2. The medical staff determines whether the bedwetting has a medical cause (other than deep sleep). If there is a medical problem, proper treatment begins.
3. If there is no evident medical problem, the family decides whether to undergo the Try for Dry program, pursue other treatments, or do nothing.

The reason that wetting has not merited true medical status is that traditional treatments have either not shown reliable remissions of wetting or the medical basis of the treatment was unclear. So, all too often, wetting problems are discounted as nonmedical. Also, the treatment of wetting problems is not regularly taught in medical schools or residency training programs.

Because of these facts, it is not surprising that the doctor's stock answer might have been: "Don't worry, she'll outgrow it." To the family, this advice seems to imply that wetting in fact does not cause any real difficulties and that nothing can be done to stop it.

We believe that wetting disorders are a legitimate medical problem. Eventually, researchers will come to decipher the medical basis of wetting. In the meantime, doctors and parents must take care of children's needs without this clear knowledge.

Mothers Know Best

When we began focusing on the treatment of childhood wetting problems in our practice, we routinely performed a variety of tests on our patients to rule out three known primary causes of wetting: (1) urine infections, (2) kidney disorders, and (3) bladder and urethra disorders. Occasionally the tests were misleading; so when a child continued to wet despite normal test results and treatment, we performed a visual test of the bladder, called a cystoscopy. Eventually we recognized a basic phenomenon: the more tests we did, the more normal results we got. So we decided to minimize testing in our approach.

We came to realize that in the field of childhood wetting, as in so many other pediatric specialties, mothers have the answers. We simply had to learn what to listen for and how to interpret what we heard. Mothers regularly hit us over the head with solid information. Their observations about their child's wetting behavior usually related to at least one of four causes: (1) deep sleep, (2) small bladder capacity, (3) irregular defecation, and (4) dietary sensitivities. Some told us that they had trouble waking their otherwise well-adjusted and healthy child for school in the morning. Others described their difficult car trips, how they had

A "RIGHT" TO BE DRY?

Should every family choose treatment for their children who wet? Or does it make more sense for a family to wait, even though it may take months, perhaps years, for a child to outgrow the problem? To answer these questions logically, one must judge the overall benefit to the child in relation to the risks and costs of treatment. That's a judgment that ultimately falls to each family.

Although wetting conditions do tend to resolve themselves spontaneously (about 15 percent per year), we do not recommend delaying evaluation and treatment. We believe that all children at least have a right to be evaluated. Then, after an initial evaluation by a qualified medical professional, a family should decide how to proceed. For those who choose treatment, an appropriate plan that meets the family's needs can be devised for any child who is able to understand and follow instructions—usually after age two. Wetting treatments can be a catalyst for change: in a matter of months, an appropriate dryness program can help stop the wetting that might have taken a child years to outgrow.

Keep in mind that it is rare for wetting to be caused by structural deformities ("birth defects") or by major psychological conditions. As we will explain in detail in Chapter 2, physiological problems such as small bladder capacity and deep sleep are the major causes of wetting in children.

to keep stopping at rest stops every hour so their children could go to the bathroom. We heard about children who tended to be constipated or who defecated only twice a week; only rarely did we hear that children without wetting difficulties—whom we were evaluating for other conditions—had such a constipation problem. Finally, mothers themselves noted that when their children ate or drank certain things, their wetting worsened.

In developing our scheme to cure bedwetting, we devised a treatment approach for each of these four factors:

1. **Deep sleep.** When asleep, the child wears a moisture-sensitive alarm that sounds at the first drops of urine.

2. **Small bladder capacity.** The child takes a medication that lessens bladder contractions that are "too strong" and also lessens the feeling of urgency to urinate. (For day wetting, the medication helps give the child more time to get to the toilet after he feels the need to urinate.)

3. **Irregular defecation.** The child follows a toileting regimen to encourage daily morning bowel movements.

4. **Diet.** By following an "elimination" diet, the child and family try to identify and then eliminate foods that may hinder bladder control.

(More recently, we have also become concerned about the roles of attention deficit hyperactivity disorder and sleep apnea in bedwetting. We discuss these conditions in more detail in Chapter 2.)

In the case of your child's wetting, you may decide to address only one or two of the four major symptoms if you believe your child, say, sleeps deeply and is constipated but shows no other signs of trouble. As you will see in Chapter 4, it is essential to know your child's sleeping, toileting, and eating habits in order to devise an ideal plan to get to dry.

What Lies Ahead

We have based the recommendations in this book on our own experience treating many hundreds of children with enuresis and incontinence. As you will begin to see in Chapter 4, you and your child will attack the wetting problem in four phases:

1. Observe and record by diary your child's bodily functions, including when and what she eats and drinks and when and how much and how often she urinates, and how often she moves her bowels. (Chapter 4)

2. In consultation with your family health-care provider, and using the information you have recorded, determine the likely causes of your child's wetting. (Chapter 4)

3. Choose and implement a treatment plan that targets those particular causes. Also enlist your child's cooperation. (Chapters 5 and 6)

4. Help your child follow through with the plan, working through relapses and complications, until the wetting stops. (Chapters 7, 8, and 9)

Our scheme is *multi-modal;* that is, it incorporates a number of treatment options into each child's plan, based on a particular child's needs. It relies not on a single, universal technique or device, but on a repertoire of several methods. You—with help from your doctor—choose which combination of treatments to use, according to the specific factors that contribute to your child's wetting.

Summary

In the early days of our practice, we were dismayed to find that some children had wetting problems that resisted our interventions, even after they tried to address each of the four most common contributing factors. Then we began monitoring the children more closely, making sure, for example, the alarm was being used properly. We found that some parents, instead of rousing the child themselves when the alarm went off, were waiting for the child to get himself up. In other families, we found that the child needed the alarm sensor to be sewn closer to the spot where the bladder empties (lower on the underpants for girls and higher on the underpants for boys). Once we fine-tuned the treatments for these children, very few "hard cases" were left.

The few remaining children who we could not get dry visited our psychologist, at which point we found that the children simply did not follow the program well enough. Some younger children were opposed to wearing the alarm; some older children were secretly eating foods that seemed to contribute to their wetting. We only rarely found significant psychological disturbance in any child or family.

This leads us to one all-important point:

Children who wet, and their families, are normal.

As you read and talk about this book with your child, please emphasize that message to him and keep it in mind yourself. Children acquire so much of their outlook and behavior from their parents. When your child sees your optimism, he is more likely to share it.

The Jewish folk lullaby "Yankele" recognizes the frustration that bedwetting causes even in a happy, attentive family:

> Go to sleep, my Yankele, my sweet one,
> Your dark eyes please close,
>
> A boy who already has all his teeth,
> your mother still has to sing to sleep,
>
> . . .
>
> A boy who'll be a clever groom-to-be
> Why must you sleep so wet as if in a lake?

As you and your family work together to understand and ultimately overcome your child's wetting, we encourage you to maintain a supportive, loving environment in your home. Your affection, your optimism, and your perseverance will help carry him toward his goal.

PART ONE

Understanding the Problem

CHAPTER 1

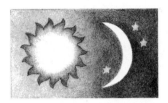

Wetting Matters:
An Overview

O UR FIRST objective in this chapter is to clarify the terminology we will be using throughout this book. As with so many medical subjects, some names and terms associated with wetting may seem confusing or ambiguous to those unfamiliar with them. You may want to refer to this section, as well as the glossary in the back of the book, as you continue reading.

Enuresis or Incontinence?

The medical terms most commonly used to describe wetting disorders are *enuresis* and *incontinence*. Lay people and doctors tend to use these words interchangeably to mean "lack of good bladder control." In this book and in our practice, we choose between these two terms very carefully, as they distinguish between two different reasons for wetness.

- We define *enuresis* as wetting caused by problems that do not need surgical correction (which is the case in about 99 percent of children who wet).
- We define *incontinence* as wetting caused by problems that *do* need surgical intervention (which is the case in about 1 to 3 percent of children who wet).

Why do we need two different words when the results are equally wet? Because our terminology should remind us that some wetting problems can be caused by "birth defects," such as a problem with the kidneys, bladder, ureters, or urethra. In children who are diagnosed as incontinent, fixing the defect with surgery is usually necessary to stop the wetting.

In our terms, children who are diagnosed with enuresis wet despite having a normally formed urinary tract (see Figure 1-1 and Figure 1-2 on pages 6 and 7). In other words, their kidneys, ureters, bladder, and urethra have no malformations, but there is a problem with bladder function—that is, a problem with how the bladder does its job of storing and expelling urine.

When we diagnose enuresis (not incontinence) as the cause of a child's wetting condition, then we recommend that the child consistently follow the treatment program described in this book. If enuresis is indeed the problem, we expect that the child will become dry after a few months of treatment.

If, however, we diagnose a child with enuresis but he does not become dry after following the dryness regimen for a few months, we usually suggest to the parents that we perform a more detailed medical examination. An underlying birth defect—that is, a diagnosis of incontinence—may be the explanation. Children diagnosed with incontinence wet because their urinary tract is not normally formed. Undergoing surgery is

DRIVING LESSONS

We try to come up with colorful metaphors when we talk with children, especially young ones, about controlling bodily functions. In the case of the bladder and the urinary system, we tell a child that, just as grown-ups drive cars, she drives her bladder. Automobile drivers learn how to control and operate a car just as she is learning how to control her urination.

Furthermore, when we explain the difference between enuresis and incontinence to children, we say that cars and urinary systems alike need help when things aren't working right. If the child has enuresis, her whole system may need a tune-up: the dryness program will help get her system running smoothly. If the child has incontinence, though, some parts might need to be repaired or replaced to fix the problem: simple surgery usually does the trick.

probably the only way the child will get to dry. (See Appendix C for the most common disorders associated with incontinence.)

Thus, this distinction between enuresis and incontinence is a constant reminder that if a child does not get to dry after a few months of treatment, incontinence may be causing the wetting. When you talk to your child or to friends and family about wetting, be sure to remember the difference between enuresis and incontinence. And explain it to other people, who probably *do not* distinguish between the two.

ENURESIS: SECONDARY OR PRIMARY?

It is important to note the difference between primary and secondary enuresis when evaluating your child or discussing this problem with your physician or health-care provider. Although a mother may consider her son toilet trained because he wears

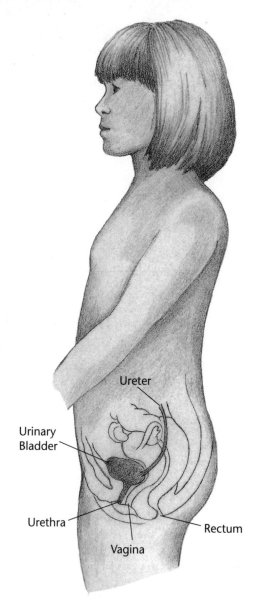

Ureter

Urinary
Bladder

Urethra

Vagina

Rectum

Figure 1-1. The normally formed urinary tract in girls

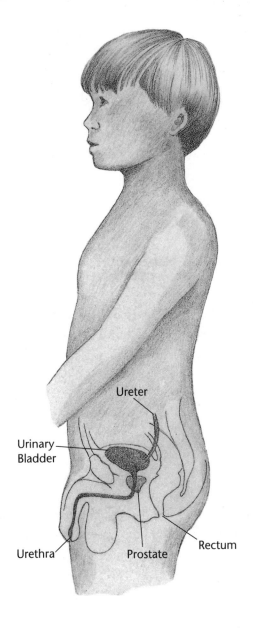

Figure 1-2. The normally formed urinary tract in boys

underpants, not diapers, if the child has always wet right through his clothes, he has in fact never been toilet trained.

When a child has never been dry—that is, if she has always wet by day or night on a regular basis without sustaining dryness for more than six months—that child is said to have *primary enuresis.* This describes the majority of children who wet.

If a child has achieved dryness for at least six months some-time in her life but then begins to wet again, she is said to have *secondary enuresis.* This occurs in 3 to 8 percent of children be-tween five and thirteen years old.

POPULAR EXPRESSIONS

In everyday language, wetting problems usually fall into three categories:

- **Bedwetting.** The greatest number of children who wet experi-ence what is commonly called *bedwetting.* It may also be called *night wetting* or *sleep wetting.* Doctors refer to this type of wet-ting as *nocturnal wetting* or *nocturnal enuresis,* both of which mean "to wet at night." If your child wets at night, you might have noticed that she usually urinates during periods of deep sleep and is not easily awakened. Youngsters who bedwet may also wet during daytime naps. The common mechanism be-hind the wetting is not the "bed," it is the deep sleep, by day or by night, that interferes with a child's perception of an impending bladder contraction. Because children who wet cannot easily inhibit their contraction well, they wet, whether in a car seat during a nap or in bed at night. Some children who bedwet may also experience during the daytime symp-toms of urgency, frequency, and daytime dampness.
- **Day wetting.** Some children lose bladder control only during the day. We call that condition *day wetting* or *diurnal enuresis.*

Like bedwetting, day wetting happens when a child has poor bladder control. The condition can be mild enough to cause slight dampening of underwear or pants or severe enough to result in soaked clothing.

- **Giggle wetting.** An infrequent kind of day wetting, which incidentally seems to be more prevalent in girls, is *giggle wetting.* Children who giggle-wet do so while laughing, giggling, or being tickled. Though the name seems funny, children with this condition can feel tremendous embarrassment and shame in front of their friends.

Your child may experience one, two, or all three types of wetting. But, no matter what type of wetting problem he has, there are treatment options available. As the illustration of the sun and the moon at the beginning of each chapter symbolizes, we can treat wetting that occurs by day and/or by night. Your intimate knowledge of your child's wetting pattern will be your first tool in choosing the most appropriate treatments for him. (You will record this and other important information on our questionnaire when you read Chapter 4.)

Making Sure You Need This Book

School-age children who lack bladder control are almost always unhappy with the condition, yet they may not readily admit it. It is most likely that you, the child's parent, are also unhappy—as well as siblings and other family members. And although no one should be embarrassed by wetting—no more than someone with asthma or diabetes would be embarrassed by his or her condition—children who wet are often stigmatized as "babies" or "bedwetters" or worse. Wetting can also be disruptive: after just a few nights of interrupted sleep, because pajamas and sheets need changing, parents and children begin to show the strain.

Before we go any further, though, let's be sure that your child needs to undergo the treatment plans described in this book. First, if you haven't already done so, try some or all of the following tactics; they should help anyone sleep through the night without having to use the toilet.

- Promote the idea of dryness during daily activities, and build mental cues that reinforce the idea. For example, read child-oriented books on the subject with your child, talk to him about the benefits of being dry (such as going on sleepovers), and try to create a positive environment for getting to dry.
- Make sure your child is getting plenty of rest. An overtired child is more likely to sleep so deeply that he will have more trouble "learning" dryness.
- Keep your child from drinking too much liquid before bed.
- Encourage your child to urinate in the toilet before going to bed every night.
- Avoid letting your older child sleep in diapers, Pull-Ups, or other absorbent undergarments (see page 127).
- Once or twice a night, carry the child from bed to the toilet to urinate (see "Scheduled Lifting: An Alternative Approach," page 116).

If your child's wetting persists despite these efforts, then you will benefit from the treatments described in this book.

A Few Words of Advice

While you are reading the next few chapters, becoming more familiar with the causes of your child's wetting and preparing to begin the remedies described in Part Two, keep in mind the following suggestions:

Reduce the Stress in Your Family's Life. Just after the arrival of a new baby is not the time to begin trying to change your child's long-term wetting problem. It is important that other stressors be kept to a minimum during treatment—both for your sake and for your child's. He will need extra attention and understanding. Because of the focus and commitment required by the program, other major projects competing for your time and attention will most likely have to be put aside for a time. To try halfheartedly to get to dry and then give up prematurely would be more discouraging to you and more devastating to your child than simply doing nothing. So to the extent possible, make getting to dry your top priority.

Choose Optimism. Our children imitate us in so many ways—the way we dress, the way we talk, the things we laugh at. When the subject is wetting, your child will take her cues from you. If you present the program with a positive attitude and lots of encouragement, you're sowing the seeds of success. If you react calmly and confidently during difficult times, you'll be sending your child a clear message: We can handle this together. This book will show you how.

Enlist the Support of Others. Neither you nor your child would feel comfortable broadcasting details of his wetting problem to the entire neighborhood, but, depending on your circumstances, certain key people should be told. Teachers, for example, need to be aware if your child wets during the day so that they can give your child easy access to the toilet. You may find support in speaking to another family that has experienced bedwetting. Remember, though, your child is probably sensitive about his wetting and would prefer to keep it private. Extended family members and others who care for your child when he might wet, such as grandparents and babysitters, also need to know about your child's wetting problem.

Simplify Clean-up. Optimism and determination go a long way, but there's no denying the benefits of a good mattress pad. Use absorbent bedding with a plastic mattress cover. (See "Clearing the Air" on the opposite page, and see Appendix D for a directory of product suppliers.)

Summary

We hope this chapter has equipped you with a basic understanding of bedwetting and the types of wetting problems. You should now know what to do to prepare yourself and your child for getting to dry.

Keep in mind the following essential points, all of which we have discussed in this chapter:

1. We classify a wetting problem as either (a) enuresis, which can be corrected without surgery, or (b) incontinence, which requires surgery to correct the wetting. Most children who wet have enuresis, not incontinence, and can attain dryness without surgical intervention.

2. Children with primary enuresis have never had adequate control of their bladder. Children with secondary enuresis have had a period of bladder control lasting at least six consecutive months at some time in their lives.

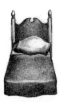

CLEARING THE AIR

Urine-soaked clothing and bed linens tend to retain strong odors. Odor can be a particular problem when children wet by day, because the urine generally has plenty of time to soak into clothing. When urine leaks onto clothes, it activates bacterial spores that remain in the clothes after normal washing. These spores are the likely culprit when children smell of urine even though they just changed into newly laundered clothes. Ordinary chlorine bleach and laundry detergent do not seem to kill the spores. If the spores are not destroyed, they may reactivate the next time they come in contact with urine and multiply more rapidly than before, causing an even stronger odor.

If you find that regular laundering does not remove the smell from your child's clothes or bedding, try soaking the soiled articles in an enzyme bleach or borax solution prior to washing. These agents are more effective at getting rid of the spores and so also the odor.

3. There are three popular names that apply to both enuresis and incontinence: (a) bedwetting, (b) day wetting, and (c) giggle wetting.

4. It is very important that you try to reduce the stress in your family's life and find workable, practical ways to cope with the chores and routines necessitated by handling your child's wetting.

You are now ready to proceed to Chapter 2. In addition to a description of normal bladder function, we present more details about how children normally become dry and what may cause wetting to persist. Then, in Chapter 3, we reveal the truth behind the most common myths about wetting, and we describe some of the ways that children respond to their problem.

Questions and Answers

Q: *There's a lot of advice out there about bedwetting—from my mother-in-law to other bedwetting books to Internet Websites. What's different about the Try for Dry approach?*

A: The approach we use in our practice, the same one offered in this book, distinguishes itself from existing treatments for bedwetting in at least four ways:

1. It is the only comprehensive, *medically based,* organized approach that deals with wetting problems by day, by night, or both.
2. The treatments we recommend are *multi-modal;* that is, they consist of several remedies working together. The result is wetting stops sooner and the effects last longer than when single modes of treatment are used.
3. The cost of treatment is minimized, because we focus on the use of a one-time-purchase enuresis alarm and inexpensive medication.
4. Articles describing the treatment success of our program have been published in medical journals.

Q: *My four-and-a-half-year-old son has recently started wetting only at night after being completely dry since age three. Out of the last nine nights, he has wet seven. We simply change him and put him back to bed. Any suggestions?*

A: It is worthwhile to be sure that there is not a medical reason for your boy's return to bedwetting, the most common being a urine infection. If your doctor reports that your child has a normal physical examination and that a sample of urine checked in the office does not show infection, simply putting him back into Pull-Ups is one way to temporarily deal with the situation. Depending on how aggressive you want to be with the problem, you may choose to (1) see if you can figure out about what time he wets, and then lift him to the toilet before this happens; (2) reduce *mildly* the amount of liquids he's allowed to drink after dinner; and (3) take note of whether he's having a bowel movement daily. If not, try a little apple juice. These few suggestions should get you started while you read more about our program.

Q: *Do I really need to visit the doctor about bedwetting? Can't I just follow the instructions in this book without spending the time and money on a doctor's visit?*

A: Statistically, it's unlikely that the doctor will find a problem during a physical examination of your child, and your child's urine tests will probably be normal. So, it's likely that he has enuresis, not incontinence; that is, he's unlikely to need surgery to correct an anatomical defect that is causing the wetting. Nevertheless, a visit to the doctor is important so that you can rule out surgery and also for several other reasons. As you will learn in Chapter 6, the use of the prescription drug oxybutynin (Ditropan) is helpful in attaining dryness. Your doctor will need to prescribe this if you choose to try the medication. In addition, you may appreciate the support of your doctor—and your child may be more motivated to change with a doctor's involvement—as you follow the procedures in this book.

Chapter 2

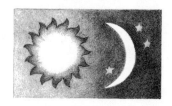

The Physiology
of Wetting

ONE OF THE first milestones on the path to dryness—for you and for your child—is gaining understanding. You need to know (1) why most children do not wet, (2) why some children do wet, and, most important, (3) what might be the causes of your own child's wetting problem. Only after you have gained real insight into your child's unique condition can you successfully choose and undertake a treatment plan.

In this chapter, we explain how children normally acquire bladder control and what we think prevents some children from mastering this skill. Next, we present a summary of the causes of and contributors to wetting problems, which range from deep sleep to diet. This is the general information you will need so that, in consultation with your doctor, you can begin to implement the dryness techniques described in Chapters 5 and 6.

Normal Development of Bladder Function

Newborn babies have no bladder control: they reflexively release urine from the bladder approximately every two hours, or about twelve to sixteen times a day. As a *newborn's* bladder fills with urine, it stretches until it reaches full capacity (about two ounces). Then receptors in the muscle that lines the bladder wall (called the *bladder detrusor* muscle) cause it to contract by reflex, expelling the urine. At this stage of development, babies are unaware of urinating; the brain plays a very minor role, if any, in initiating and stopping the release of urine. In newborns, urinating is a simple muscle reflex.

By about the end of *infancy,* because nervous system connections between the bladder and the brain work better, children begin to sense bladder fullness while awake. As soon as children come to recognize this sensation, they can start developing their ability to inhibit the release of urine. They do so by contracting the muscle situated at the neck of the bladder (called the *bladder sphincter* muscle).

By the time children reach *toddlerhood,* that is, between two and four years old, they can be expected to have control of their bladder during the day. By now, they likely have the muscle strength and coordination to master urinary control. They also are motivated by parental expectations and rewards, and by the satisfaction of emulating their toilet-trained peers. Usually by four years of age, children can stop a bladder contraction when they want to as well as initiate urination when they want to. This ability is called *volitional bladder control.*

Children older than five years—that is, *youths*—typically maintain volitional bladder control by day. We say that such a child has achieved daytime *urinary continence.* The child has learned that when he does not want to urinate, he must (1) in-

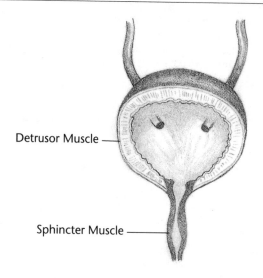

Detrusor Muscle ——

Sphincter Muscle ——

Figure 2-1. The urinary bladder

hibit a contraction of the bladder detrusor muscle and (2) actively contract the bladder sphincter muscle. In addition, the child considers how much he has drunk, where any nearby bathrooms are, and so on. When it is convenient and socially acceptable, he will permit his bladder to empty by (1) contracting the bladder detrusor while (2) relaxing the bladder sphincter. Sometimes, a little grunt helps push out the urine and get the urination started.

Urinary control normally comes first during the day while a child is awake, then during naps, and finally at night. Children usually achieve bowel continence—that is, the willful control and release of stool—before they have achieved urinary continence. Bowel control ordinarily develops first at night, then during the day.

The reasons why children get to dry at night on their own are unknown. So, setting an age at which children "should" be dry is arbitrary. Most authorities assume that the child will outgrow the wetting and give the conventional advice: "Don't worry about wetting until after she's five years old." Others say, "Wait until she's seven." Still others say, "Wait until she's nine." Our approach is very different. We regard wetting as a condition that can be addressed at almost *any* age after infancy, with treatments tailored for specific age groups.

How Children Normally Achieve Daytime Dryness

During waking hours, children who stay dry can do so because the normal physiology just described works well for them. In particular, when children begin to acquire the ability to sense what their bladder is telling them—that is, an impending release of urine—they initiate the natural process of developing dryness: they concentrate on the coming contraction. A child may stare off into space as he forms a mental concept of the bladder activity. His face and cheeks may turn red while he tries to inhibit the bladder contraction. Usually, when a parent sees a child doing this, the parent initiates toilet training (or the child may walk to the bathroom himself). When such natural behavior is supplemented with regular trips to the bathroom—what we call *scheduled voiding*—a child will begin to stay dry all day.

Some other behaviors signal a child's readiness for toilet training:

- **Dancing on their toes.** By contracting their pelvic muscles as much as possible, children try to prevent the bladder contraction from expelling the urine.
- **Squatting.** When children squat and push the heel of one foot into their bottom—the anus or perineum—the heel acts like a cork on the bladder, so it is physically impossible for the

bladder contraction to empty the bladder. Some children accomplish this by sitting on the edge of a stool or chair.

- **Making an announcement.** Some children will tell their parents—and anyone else around—that they are going "pee-pee" in their diaper or training pants. The child's newfound awareness of this sensation can be a child's first motivator toward toilet training.

Parents who have learned to read the external signs of their child's internal body functions—the contractions of the bladder sphincter and detrusor—can reinforce urinary continence with rewards (such as praise, hugs, or stickers). Children who are motivated to be dry and who have developed the motor skills to coordinate toileting tasks (getting to the toilet in time, lowering their pants and underpants, urinating, wiping if appropriate, then raising their underwear and pants) are quick to show daytime dryness. Still, dryness develops faster for some than others, and usually for girls before boys.

There are many natural and artificial obstacles to acquiring daytime urinary continence. Children who drink too much, have small bladder capacity, or have not achieved complete bowel continence, for example, may take longer to develop daytime dryness. Also, when parents are inconsistent in rewarding dryness or unresponsive to their child's signals, progress may be slower than normal.

How Children Normally Achieve Nighttime Dryness

We understand little about how children normally become dry at night. We do know that motivating children to stay dry by building mental cues does help. Parents can do a number of

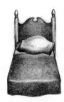

STRENGTH IN NUMBERS

Eighty-five percent of five-year-olds have complete bladder control, all day and all night. That leaves 15 percent of them with wet pants or a wet bed—or both—whether occasionally or every day. So four or five children in a class of thirty kindergartners are battling some problem with wetting. That amounts to about five million American children who suffer bedwetting at any given time.

Unfortunately, all too often a child feels as if he is the only one in the world who wets. Obviously, no five-year-old who has trouble staying dry is alone. Whether they suffer from chronic ongoing wetting or occasional relapses, lots of young children are faced with the same problem.

things to help children attain nighttime dryness, including the following:

- Start a reward system (a sticker chart for dry nights, with a prize given for a certain number of stickers).
- Prevent the child from overdrinking.
- Encourage the child to urinate completely before going to sleep at night.
- Build the habit of staying dry overnight by lifting the child to the toilet at least once during the night.

It is still a mystery how children inhibit bladder contractions while they sleep. Children wet at night for a wide variety of reasons, but they all boil down to two: While children who wet are asleep, (1) they cannot wake themselves when their bladder signals that it is full and (2) they cannot prevent a bladder contraction. Once they can perform these two actions, they will stay dry at night.

Likely Causes of Wetting

In order to find the appropriate likely solutions to your child's wetting problem, you need to consider what medical or psychological factors might be at work.

Remember that we use the word *enuresis* to refer to a wetting problem apparently not caused by a physical defect. So, if not the result of a "birth defect," what else might be causing the wetting? Perhaps a better way to ask the question is, "What is preventing your older child from outgrowing the wetting that we regard as normal in infants?"

In addition, if we accept the fact that most children who bedwet can control their bladder by day, we should ask, "How can a child control her bladder by day but not by night?"

To answer this latter question, consider the three skills children must master in order to achieve *daytime* bladder control:

1. The ability to *sense* when a bladder contraction is imminent
2. The ability to *voluntarily* inhibit the bladder muscle from contracting
3. The ability to contract their urine-holding muscle (the bladder sphincter—the one we rely on after the movie has ended and the theater restroom is packed)

The key words here are the intuitive functions of *sensation* and *volition*. If we agree that the common thread of these functions is awareness, then we conclude that children who bedwet sleep so deeply that they may not have the skill to perform these functions.

ONE BOY'S PROBLEM

Let's take the case of a boy we'll call Denton, who bedwets occasionally. *During sleep,* Denton can sense an impending bladder contraction, inhibit the contraction, and possibly actively tighten his bladder sphincter, and so stay dry.

Alternatively, if Denton's bladder is very full and he is not sleeping very deeply, then he may arouse himself, go to the toilet and urinate, and return to bed. The key word here is *arouse*. Children who do not wet the bed can wake themselves to use the toilet at night.

Consider the differences in the following scenarios:

Saturday. Denton, at his own birthday party in the afternoon, eats his fill of cake and *overdrinks* soda and juice. After dinner he continues to celebrate with cake and soda with his family. That night he gets up a few times to urinate in the toilet but otherwise he sleeps soundly—in a dry bed.

Why? Despite all the liquids he consumed, Denton stayed dry because he has acquired the ability to wake himself when he senses that his bladder is full—*if he's not sleeping too deeply.* Denton went to bed at nine and then awakened to urinate in the toilet at typical intervals of time: first around eleven, then again at two, and finally again at five.

Monday. After school, Denton plays a Little League game in the afternoon and comes home exhausted. After rushing through dinner, he does his homework and goes off to bed. At two in the morning, Denton wets his bed.

Why? The stress of the game? Fear of a poor grade in school? No. Probably because he went to bed so overtired that he slept too deeply to sense his bladder's fullness.

Sunday. Denton pitches the last four innings of the Little League playoff game. Between innings, he gulps down cans and cans of sports drinks. Denton's team plays poorly and ultimately loses 9–4. That night Denton bedwets.

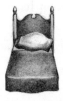

A FAMILY AFFAIR

If there is a child who wets in your family, probe your own family tree for a history of wetting: in most cases you will not have to search very far. A recent study indicated that there is a genetic predisposition associated with nighttime wetting. Statistically, a child's chance of being wet is 40 percent if one parent wet as a child; it increases to 70 percent if both parents wet as children. So the fact that a child bedwets may be just as natural as having the parents' brown eyes or blond hair. This "hard wiring," of course, does not prevent children from controlling and ending their wetting. The genetic evidence just further substantiates the idea that wetting is essentially a physiological problem, and certainly not the result of bad parenting or laziness.

Why? Ah-ha, you say, he was upset! Perhaps, but a stronger possibility is a combination of factors: he was overtired, so he slept too deeply, and he drank too much, thus overloading his limited ability to wake up to urinate.

DENTON'S CASE illustrates an important principle: whether a child wets only occasionally (like Denton) or routinely, the same causes are likely to blame. For all children who wet, we need to consider what circumstances may impede their normal process of "outgrowing" their bedwetting.

In the past, bedwetting was attributed to an "immature nervous system." We prefer to avoid the word *immature* and its negative connotations. We believe it to be just as correct to think of a child who bedwets as having not yet developed the control to coordinate the functions of inhibiting a bladder contraction, tightening the bladder sphincter, and waking up enough to get himself to the toilet. If the child also has to deal with small functional bladder capacity (see page 26) or sensitivity to common foods or beverages, or bowels so sluggish that they press on his bladder, then maintaining urinary control becomes even harder to do. On top of these complications, if his family or friends make him feel ashamed, then achieving dryness becomes an enormous task. In this chapter and the next, we discuss each of these factors in detail.

DEEP SLEEP

"William sleeps so heavily, the train that passes behind our house doesn't budge him!"

Parents often wonder how failure of arousal from sleep influences bedwetting. The answer is, if the sound of a freight train doesn't wake the child, then the call of a full bladder about to empty itself won't either.

Although wetting may occur in all stages of the sleep cycle, one factor is consistently associated with bedwetting: the intensity of sleep. Almost universally, parents report that their children who wet by night sleep more heavily than siblings who don't bedwet, or more heavily than what the parents would consider average. In what some parents have called "dead sleep," children move around very little, are not easily roused from their slumber, and, when awakened, are often disoriented.

Among traditional medical scientists, however, deep sleep—or perhaps more correctly "failure of arousal"—is a controversial explanation for wetting problems. Most scientists approach a problem by defining the characteristics of its parts. In other words, scientists need to quantify what they observe. We have measurement systems for weight, for height, even for such amorphous characteristics as intelligence. This ability to measure is the foundation for scientific investigation.

In the case of wetting problems, scientists want to measure the relationship between deep sleep and wetting. One recent study attempted to do so by monitoring the sleep patterns of fifteen enuretic boys and eighteen boys who did not wet. The researchers, at the University of Ottawa, first allowed the boys to sleep uninterrupted for two nights, so they could adjust to the monitoring equipment. Before the third night's sleep, all the boys put on headphones and were instructed to press a button three times and say "I am awake" upon hearing a tone as they slept. The result: the children who did not bedwet responded more often to the tone than children who did wet. The enuretic boys awoke only 8.5 percent of the time, while the nonenuretic boys awoke 39.6 percent of the time. This simple study supports the generally accepted concept that children who wet at night are oblivious to everything—whether it's a tone ringing in their ear or their bladder signaling its fullness.

In the Try for Dry program, though—at least until scientists can reach consensus—we take our cue from mothers' and fathers' observations of their own children.

SMALL FUNCTIONAL BLADDER CAPACITY

"My toilet-trained five-year-old can pee out more at one time than my ten-year-old, who can't stop bedwetting."

Another factor consistently found in youths with primary nocturnal enuresis is small functional bladder capacity. How does small bladder capacity make it harder to get to dry? Think of toilet training as a learning process. Learning of any kind is more difficult when there are distractions. It's harder to concentrate on a book when the TV is on. Likewise, we can't expect children to pay attention for an impending bladder contraction—that is, to monitor their feeling or urgency—while they are engrossed in a TV show or a computer game.

We consider small bladder capacity to be an additional distractor. Children with small bladder capacity have less forewarning of the need to urinate: they feel more urgency. So, for kids who wet easily because they have this feeling of urgency and cannot hold more than a small amount of urine, learning dryness is harder.

In Chapter 4, we will show you how to determine your child's functional bladder capacity, which is defined as the largest volume of urine at which the bladder can function, that is, hold its contents. It is also the largest amount that the bladder can empty at one time, as measured by monitoring a child's voiding over a three-day period. (See pages 74–75 and pages 80–81 for instructions on keeping and understanding a *voiding diary*.)

The functional bladder capacity in children who do not wet usually increases as the child gets older. In general, children who do not bedwet have normal bladder capacity for their age, roughly calculated in ounces by adding two to their age in years. So, for example, a normally functioning seven-year-old girl would be expected to have a bladder capacity of nine ounces.

This measurement is important because if your child's bladder holds less urine on average than that of other children her age and size, she may have problems getting to dry at night. It is also possible that she may have trouble holding enough urine to get to the toilet during the day.

"Mom, I just couldn't get there in time!"

Some children who bedwet may also experience daytime symptoms of (1) urgency, (2) increased frequency, and (3) damp underpants. About 25 percent of children who bedwet show these three daytime symptoms that go along with a reduced functional bladder capacity. We believe that small bladder capacity makes it harder for children to get to dry because it leaves them with a smaller margin for error.

Although small bladder capacity is not the primary cause of enuresis in most children, it is found so commonly that your doctor likely will evaluate and consider it in judging to what extent it is contributing to your child's wetting.

PROBLEMS WITH BOWEL ELIMINATION

"Some weeks, I'm afraid we'll have to spend more money paying the plumber to unstop our toilet from the huge bowel movements he has every week than on the grocery bill!"

Children with wetting problems may be affected by such bowel elimination disorders as irregular or infrequent bowel movements or constipation.

When we first began treating children who had both constipation and night wetting, we were surprised to find a connection between treatment for constipation and improved dryness. Commonly, we would correct a fecal impaction (a hard, dry plug of stool in the rectum that is removed with an enema or by manual means) and then the child's wetting would improve, or the child would get to dry using previously unsuccessful treatments. Based on what we had accidentally discovered, we began trying to change the bowel habits of children with less severe bowel problems, to see if that would help them achieve dryness.

First we found that, in response to our initial questions about bowel habits, some families of children who failed to attain dryness had not noted any bowel difficulties in their children, but in fact many of those children were experiencing bowel irregularity. After the irregularity was corrected, their bladder treatment program became very effective. While recognizing that few children are as regular as clockwork and that it's not always easy to tell exactly what children do when they go to the bathroom and close the door, we now ask detailed questions about the bowel habits of all the children we treat. The accuracy of the parents' answers to these questions is vital to their children's success in the program (see "Observing Bowel Frequency," page 82.)

Naturally, youths, preteens, and teens tend to be private about their bowel movements. Of course, you should respect your child's desire for privacy, but you should also explain to him why this information is so important. It may help to remind your child that achieving the ultimate goal—dryness—requires taking responsibility and participating in a remedy. To give up a little privacy for a few weeks in order to be dry for a lifetime is a small price to pay.

We prefer the term *regular* rather than *normal* bowel movement, because what is normal varies from one individual to the next. For some people, a normal bowel movement may be once a day in the morning. For others, a normal movement can be once every two days, and most often in the evening. On the other hand, having a regular bowel movement implies that the child is eliminating his solid waste daily, and at a regular time interval, and that the movements are comfortable for him and are not causing pain. Even if you do not believe that your child has bowel troubles, the issue needs to be considered when trying to solve his wetting problem.

THERE ARE two reasonable explanations for the influence of bowel disorders in wetting problems:

The "Numbed" Bladder. As an example, let's say a child has just fallen from her bicycle and scraped her arm. After her mother cleans the scrape on her forearm, she gives it a kiss and then rubs it gently to make it feel better. When she rubs the wound, the mother is actually stimulating inhibitory nerves, which in turn inhibit the transmissions of the nerves that convey pain. So once the rubbing starts, the child's arm feels less painful.

Similarly, when a chronically full rectum "rubs" up against the bladder wall, which is in front of it, eventually the rubbing "numbs" a child's sense of bladder fullness. This decreased sensitivity happens by day (causing day dampness) or by night (making nighttime dryness difficult).

The "Spastic" Bladder. As the bladder fills with urine, it usually expands smoothly and uniformly. If the rectum is full, however, then the bladder's expansion may be restricted, causing the bladder to respond with an automatic contraction, even though it could still hold more urine. In other words, the "spastic" bladder, as doctors call it, contracts in spasms, rather than smoothly with good control—and the result is wetting.

Signs of Constipation

Keep in mind that an irregular bowel elimination pattern is different from constipation, although both conditions, if uncorrected, can make it difficult to get to dry. If your child is constipated, his stools are hard to pass because they are large, hard, and dry; or, if there is an "impaction," he may have loose, watery diarrhea, because the impaction acts as a plug preventing the passage of anything other than this stool water. Watch for the following signs of constipation:

- **Fecal staining or "soiling" in underpants, called** *encopresis.* In such cases, the bowel holds so much stool that the bowel sphincter (or anal sphincter) gets "tired" of holding it in; when the muscle relaxes, the underpants get stained. In other circumstances, the colon may simply evacuate unpredictably.
- **Poor appetite.** Your child may say she's not hungry because

her stomach feels full. The source of her discomfort may really be a "full" colon or intestine.

- **Pain.** Your child may not feel the urge to have a bowel movement, but he may experience abdominal pain, rectal pain, or cramping before or during a bowel movement.

If your child shows any of these signs, take the necessary steps to relieve the discomfort and return your child to regularity (see "Improving Bowel Health," page 147). Bowel irregularity seems to hinder progress toward dryness in about 20 percent of enuretic children.

FOOD SENSITIVITIES

"I wonder if there's something about some of the things my daughter eats and drinks that causes the bedwetting. It's especially bad after birthday parties, when the kids have pizza, soda, cake, and ice cream."

Although scientists disagree over the details, it is clear that a person's diet can profoundly affect his or her well-being. For example, a diet low in fats can lower blood cholesterol and reduce the likelihood of heart disease. In another example, for some people who are intolerant of milk, avoiding milk products will control their diarrhea.

In the case of enuresis, there is little substantiated, scientifically proven evidence of a relationship between diet and wetting. Despite this lack of scientific proof, we have a good deal of anecdotal evidence from parents and children that avoiding certain foods or beverages may improve dryness.

We have developed a diet that is based on the observations of the families we have treated. We ask almost all the children we treat for enuresis to follow the diet, which we call the Happy

Bladder Diet, for a trial period of two weeks; it seems to help about 10 percent of those who try it. Interestingly, many of the foods and beverages that children are asked not to consume while on the Happy Bladder Diet (see page 157) are the same products that researchers in England recently proved can actually trigger bedwetting.

Some of the foods and beverages that seem to hinder progress toward dryness for some children are these:

- Milk and milk products, including ice cream and cheese
- Carbonated beverages, including colas
- Noncarbonated beverages that contain caffeine, such as coffee or tea
- Citrus fruit and citrus drinks, including oranges, grapefruit, lemons, and their juices
- Melons (especially watermelon)
- Licorice, which contains a chemical that increases urine production
- Vitamin tablets, especially those containing vitamin C

For detailed information on the Happy Bladder Diet, see "Tracking Problem Foods," page 155. Before you experiment with removing any of these foods from your child's diet, consult your doctor to make sure your child's nutrition will not suffer.

Drinking and Wetting

"He wets so much! His pajamas are wet, his sheets are wet, and his mattress is wet. You need galoshes to go into the room!"

The time of day your child drinks liquids and how much she drinks can be a factor in getting to dry. However, we do not advocate withholding fluids from any child. Children must have adequate fluid intake for proper health. Particularly in warmer climates and during summer months, the danger of dehydration is severe. Not getting enough fluids can, in hot climates, contribute to heat exhaustion and a host of serious medical problems. Also, extreme restriction of fluids in most cases appears to offer little or no benefit in the treatment of the enuresis. In fact, restricting fluids may make your child's stools dry and hard and thereby cause constipation. Parents must use their judgment and common sense to make sure their child gets enough fluids, but at the same time they need to help their child get to dry by making sure that she drinks in moderation. (See "Recreational Drinking," page 34.)

The way the body regulates how much urine the kidneys produce is, medically, very complex; in regard to wetting problems, however, we can keep our discussion simple. Daytime urine output basically reflects how much we drink. In turn, three factors influence how much fluid we void:

1. **The air temperature.** In hot environments, we sweat. The resulting water loss signals the body to produce less urine.
2. **How much salt we eat.** The more salt we eat, the more water we need to excrete. Also, when we eat salty or spicy food, we usually drink more, and so excrete more urine.
3. **The amount of naturally occurring diuretics we consume.** Some foods and beverages, such as colas and melons, are diuretics, which naturally increase the flow of urine.

For most of us, when we drink a lot of fluids, we expect that we will have to urinate within the next few hours. For some children who bedwet, they do just that. But for other children who bedwet, no matter what amount they drink during the day, their body seems to delay the urine excretion until nighttime. Observing and recording how your child's body handles fluids is an important step in selecting the right treatments for your child. We give instructions for keeping a diary of your child's fluid intake and voiding in Chapter 4.

RECREATIONAL DRINKING

Some children seem to drink a lot all day long—very often soft drinks, but also juices, milk, and water. We call such children recreational drinkers. On the one hand we say that parents should not withhold liquids from a child, but on the other hand, children should not make beverages their constant companions. Such recreational drinkers may take in more liquid than they need or than their bladder can handle.

If your child seems to drink lots of fluids, you should mention your concern to your family doctor. Your doctor can decide if a urine or blood test should be done to look for diabetes mellitus (see page 36) or if the drinking is just a habit.

Just as recreational drinkers have made a habit out of drinking, their bodies have become habituated to excreting the excess liquid as urine—either during the day or at night. In the daytime, most kids can handle the "extra" needs of their bladder. At night, though, as they sleep deeply, they do not sense their impending bladder contraction. And with extra liquid to void, there are even more contractions than usual. The result: they wet large amounts and wet more frequently during sleep.

So keep in mind that, although you should never withhold all liquids from your child—because of the danger of dehydration and other serious medical risks—you should not allow him to drink anything he wants all day long, either.

Is your child drinking too much? On average, children should consume about six 4-ounce glasses of liquid a day. A little extra liquid can help guard against constipation, but too much can be a sign of problems.

If, because of asthma or another condition, your doctor has directed a fluid-intake plan for your child, you should, of course, consult with your doctor before you make any changes in your child's drinking habits.

Other Conditions That May Result in Wetting

In this section, we explain various medical disorders that can have a direct relationship with wetting.

POLYURIA: MAKING TOO MUCH URINE AT NIGHT

"My boy must not empty his bladder when he pees. I watch him void just before bed, but he still wets the bed a half hour after he lies down!"

While we sleep, our brain normally manufactures and releases a hormone that reduces the amount of urine we produce. This hormone, called vasopressin, is an antidiuretic: *anti-* for "against," and *diuretic* for "making extra urine."

Some researchers theorize that when we lie down to sleep, our body's blood pressure temporarily increases. To counteract this effect, our body *decreases* its production of vasopressin (which brings the blood pressure back down), and as a result more urine is produced for a brief time. In children who already lack sufficient vasopressin, this explanation would account for why they may wet about one half hour after they go to sleep, even if they urinated in the toilet just before bed.

Some children with enuresis release less vasopressin than normal, according to one group of researchers. The obvious conclusion is that some children wet at night because they produce more urine than their counterparts who do not wet. However, if such children are making too much urine, why don't they wake up when their bladder is full? We still don't have a definitive answer to this question, other than the seeming association between deep sleep and bedwetting (see "Deep Sleep," page 25). In Chapter 6, we describe in detail a synthetic form of vasopressin that doctors can prescribe as part of a treatment for wetting [see "Overproduction of Urine at Night (Polyuria)," page 144].

DIABETES

Many parents whose children drink and urinate a lot worry about diabetes mellitus, a disorder in which the body does not process foods well, especially sugars, so that sugar accumulates in the bloodstream. If there is too much sugar in the blood, the kidney will make more urine, so the person with diabetes ends up drinking more to compensate for the extra urination. Your doctor can perform a routine test for sugar in the urine to see if this very unusual disorder may account for bedwetting in your child.

Another type of diabetes is diabetes insipidus. In this condition, the pituitary gland, located in the center of the brain, delivers too little of a particular hormone to the bloodstream. When the kidneys don't receive enough hormone, they do not retain water and, therefore, produce excess urine. Wetting can result.

If you suspect that your child may be diabetic, be sure to have your doctor perform a thorough examination before undertaking this or any other dryness program. If your child does indeed have either form of diabetes, the wetting can still be corrected using the techniques described in this book, once your child is receiving medical treatment (e.g., insulin) for the diabetes.

SICKLE CELL DISEASE

Children suffering from sickle cell disease may be prone to wetting problems. With this disease, normally smooth, disklike red blood cells may transform into "sickles" or crescents if there is a reduction in the amount of oxygen in the blood. Because the center of the kidney has low oxygen content, the sickle cells may appear in the kidneys' blood vessels. Since sickle cells move sluggishly in the blood vessels, the central sections of the kidney may lose their viability. Over time, this disorder may reduce the kidneys' ability to concentrate urine. As a result, children may pass large amounts of urine while asleep even if they have not drunk much liquid.

Like children with vasopressin deficits, children with sickle cell disease may also wet their beds. But why doesn't their full bladder wake them up? Again, perhaps deep sleep is the cause. In our program, children with sickle cell disease who wet at night have successfully stopped wetting by using an enuresis alarm, without resorting to supplementary hormone medicine to concentrate the urine. (See Chapter 5 for detailed instructions on using an enuresis alarm.)

URINE INFECTION

Although children may develop a urine infection because of a malformed urinary tract, most urine infections result from simple causes such as following poor hygiene (washing the genitals inadequately) or delaying using the bathroom. Children also get urine infections when their body's defenses are down—say, when they have just gotten over a cold.

Children with urine infections usually express great urgency to urinate and may need to do so more often than usual. They will literally run to the bathroom, often several times an hour. They might not get to the bathroom in time, so they may wet by day as well as by night or both. Here are some other signs to look for:

- Fatigue and irritability
- Painful urination
- Bloody or cloudy urine with a strong or foul odor
- Back pain
- Fever
- Bedsheets even wetter than usual
- Day urgency or wetting, or both, in a child who already bedwets (when not infected)

Here is how this increased urgency may happen. Urine infections can weaken the bladder functions of holding and expelling urine. The infection inflames the bladder wall, making the normally soft muscle stiff. In other words, the bladder may not distend as easily, at least temporarily, thus holding less urine than it otherwise could. Also, since an infected bladder is stiff, and so likely distends poorly, when the signal to void comes, the bladder contracts too quickly and urgently. A bladder contraction may immediately follow the urge, making children wet before they can get to the toilet.

Antibiotics usually heal urine infections, but the wetting may not stop even though the infection is gone. Some children who have shown this pattern of urgency and wetting during an infection, for some reason not yet clearly understood, may continue to show small capacity, urgency, and wetting weeks or months after the infection is gone. Once this cycle of wetting has begun, it seems that urine moisture in the genital skin and clothing fosters the growth of new bacteria, which can penetrate the body's defenses and cause yet another urine infection, repeating the cycle of infection and wetting. This situation can get even more complicated for some children who not only hold their urine back, but also come to hold their stool back, causing constipation, irregular defecation, or both (see "Problems with Bowel Elimination," page 28).

In our practice, when we evaluate children who wet and have had a urine infection sometime in the past, we find a problem in the structure of their urinary tracts about 30 percent of the time. If your child has had a urine infection, your doctor will need to decide if a pediatric urological consultation or special X-ray tests are necessary in order to treat wetting most effectively.

ATTENTION DEFICIT HYPERACTIVITY DISORDER

Ten percent of children with nighttime enuresis have attention deficit hyperactivity disorder (ADHD), and 25 percent of children who have ADHD have nighttime enuresis. At first, families of children with ADHD may be so overwhelmed by social and school problems related to the disorder that the wetting component just does not seem very serious. Parents tend to focus, understandably, on finding an effective remedy for the ADHD, and put aside their concerns over the wetting. However, once the ADHD treatments begin to show success, parents may be disappointed to find that the wetting persists. Families need to understand that the therapies aimed at ameliorating ADHD will not necessarily solve a wetting problem.

Although the reason for the association between ADHD and enuresis is unclear, in our experience it appears that children with ADHD, particularly those with daytime wetting, do not pay attention to their internal bladder cues. They are so distracted and reinforced by whatever else they are doing—watching television, playing outside, building with blocks—that they just don't stop and think that they should get up and go to the bathroom when they need to. Children with ADHD can't tear themselves away from the fun activity, which is immediately gratifying, for the task of toileting, which is not entertaining or gratifying. Some children have told us that they do initially feel the urge to urinate and then get distracted. Others seem insensitive to the fullness of their bladder.

Some children with ADHD have so much trouble completing tasks, even the task of urinating, that when they do run and use the toilet, they urinate incompletely, just long enough to relieve the pressure. Then they go back to playing—only to find that they are wet a half hour later.

We recommend that enuretic children with ADHD receive treatment for their ADHD prior to beginning treatment for the wetting, because treating the ADHD first will make the likelihood of success with the wetting program that much greater.

OTHER SLEEP DISORDERS

"He snores to wake the house."

"He grinds his teeth so much that I had to take him to the dentist."

Some children have other medical problems that may cause them to sleep poorly, which can in turn affect their ability to stay dry through the night. One common problem among children is enlarged or inflamed tonsils. In some cases, large tonsils can restrict airflow, possibly causing the child's brain to get too little oxygen. It's reasonable to believe that this lack of oxygen to the brain can impair the brain's performance and the child's ability to control normal bodily functions, including bladder control, during sleep.

Restricted airflow can lead to intermittent stopped breathing,

HELPING A CHILD TO FOCUS

One seven-year-old youngster, John, was having trouble becoming dry during the day and night using our standard program. During an interview with the family, it became clear that John was having difficulty getting his work done in school. The teacher repeatedly told John's parents that John could not sit still in class or stay in his seat, and that he blurted out answers and frequently disturbed other children. At home, he was somewhat defiant and was driving his parents crazy. After being diagnosed with ADHD, he began taking Ritalin, using an enuresis alarm (which we discuss fully in Chapter 5), and undergoing behavior modification. Not only did his behavior at school and at home improve dramatically, but John also started using the toilet more regularly and soon became completely dry first during the day and then at night.

called apnea. Aside from enlarged tonsils and adenoids, apnea can be caused by a number of other conditions. Symptoms of apnea might include irregular or noisy breathing, snoring, and teeth grinding, along with morning headaches and excessive morning thirst. Your child should be evaluated by a physician if he or she shows any of the symptoms associated with sleep apnea.

INCONTINENCE

As we explained in Chapter 1, *incontinence* refers to wetting caused by malformations of a child's urinary tract. Although they are the least common cause of wetting in children, such defects are associated with the most potential harm to a child's health. For this reason, and because the defects are curable only with surgery, children who wet sometimes undergo an evaluation by a pediatric urologist, who specializes in diagnosing and correcting such problems. Most disorders of incontinence are curable with surgery.

Incontinence likely affects between 1 and 3 percent of children who wet; children with incontinence usually have more than just routine bedwetting. They may show two or more of the following signs:

- Day wetting
- Night wetting
- Urine infection
- Blood in the urine
- A weak or intermittent urine stream (or both). In boys, the stream is so weak that they have to sit down or stand very close to the toilet to void. In girls, one can hear the stream's lack of force and intermittent nature as it hits the water in the toilet bowl.
- Continual dampness despite normal voiding
- In toddlers or youths, too frequent or too infrequent urination. (See Appendix C for further discussion of this symptom.)

Be careful not to jump to the conclusion that your child needs surgery. It is more reasonable to assume that a child will not require surgical intervention. If, after reading and following the recommendations in the rest of this book, you find that your child is not responding favorably to treatment for enuresis, and if your health-care provider recommends that you see a specialist, you may want to read Appendix C, which describes some of the most common disorders that cause incontinence.

Other Factors That May Contribute to Wetting

STRESS

Children who have never been dry—that is, those who have primary enuresis—may have difficulty becoming dry in the midst of stressful life circumstances. Daily stresses such as family conflict, problems at school, illness, or friction between the enuretic child and other children may precipitate a wet night. Also, children who have previously attained dryness may start wetting—that is, show secondary enuresis—after experiencing stressful life events, some of which are mentioned below.

A recent study showed that children who have four or more stressful life events in a year are two-and-a-half times more likely to develop secondary enuresis than children who do not experience any stressful events. In addition, the researchers found that children who first gained bladder control after age five were more than three times more likely to develop secondary enuresis—without additional stress. Children who attained bladder control after age five and experienced four or more stressful life events were eight times more likely to develop secondary enuresis.

When a stressful situation develops—which could be as ordinary as the birth of a new sibling or a move to a new home, or as devastating as sexual abuse or the death of a parent—a child now dry at night but prone to wetting problems may begin to wet under the new circumstances. Perhaps the child normally has mild deep sleep, a slightly small functional bladder capacity, some food sensitivities, and mild bowel disturbances but does not wet. When she is exposed to new, stressful circumstances, perhaps a new school, or her parents' divorce, or the death of a pet, wetting may occur transiently. The transient episodes, however, may breed more wetting and lead to a renewed pattern of frequent wetting. This phenomenon of "spiraling" illness may also be noted when a child with a urine infection develops more urine infections, or a child with a cold develops an ear infection, which then leads to bronchitis, and so on.

Left untreated, the isolated wetting episodes may stop spontaneously, but isolated wetting events can become a habit even after the precipitating stress has disappeared.

Some children do work out their stress, and yet the wetting habit persists. We can break this pattern of wetting not only by addressing whatever stressful circumstances remain, but also by dealing with all of the child's predisposing factors (deep sleep, small bladder size, food sensitivities, and bowel irregularity—see Chapter 4).

Keep in mind that even the best treatment program may fail if the parents are too distracted by a situation at home (such as a new baby) to follow it through. As we will see in the next chapter, choosing the right time to begin treatment can be crucial.

REINFORCEMENT OF WETTING

When you do something that increases or maintains a certain behavior in your child, psychologists say you are *reinforcing* that behavior. For example, a child who gets to sleep in his parents' bed after he wets his own bed is in effect rewarded, or reinforced, for wetting. Parents reinforce their child's wetting when they give a lot of positive or negative attention to the child as a result of the wetting. Negative attention can be reinforcing for a child who feels that his parents notice him only when he does something wrong. A parent who makes a big show of sympathy for the child—or conversely, reprimands the child—because of his wetting problems may unknowingly reinforce the wetting.

Parents need to consider whether their own reactions and responses to the child's enuresis may be contributing to the child's wetting. The next time your child wets, observe your reaction to the situation, both your emotional state and your behavior. How do you feel? What do you say to your child? One way to avoid the reinforcement trap is to react calmly and neutrally to wetting

STRESS: COMPLICATION OR CAUSE OF WETTING?

Researchers in one recent study concluded that a variety of psychosocial factors were *not related* to the age at which children attained nighttime dryness. These irrelevant factors include family social background (including the family's educational level and the child's birth order), stressful life events in the family, the number of changes of parental figures, and changes in home residence.

These findings regarding stress and changes in the family are inconsistent with other research we write about in this chapter, which just goes to show how difficult it is to pinpoint a sole cause of wetting. There is no consistent proof that stress does or does not cause wetting. In cases where wetting happens after a stressful event occurs, the mechanism by which the stress initiates the wetting is not understood. Wetting may be complicated by, but is not solely caused by, stress in the family. We do recognize, however, that stress can not only hinder us from doing our everyday tasks, but also lead to inconsistent follow-through in a dryness program.

episodes. If you find it hard to keep your emotions in check when faced with another wet bed, take a few minutes away from the situation to regain control. The less attention you draw to the problem, the less likely it is that you will reinforce the wetting.

Once again, note that psychological issues do not necessarily cause the wetting, but, once the pattern is established, they may prolong it.

Summary

In this chapter, we have touched on the primary explanations of why wetting, especially bedwetting, might happen. Here are some of the most important points to remember:

1. No single cause is responsible for all bedwetting. Thus, no single treatment can cure wetting, either.

2. We do not fully understand why, but most children who wet by night are deep sleepers.

3. Besides deep sleep, the major causes of wetting are (a) small functional bladder capacity, (b) bowel elimination disorders, and (c) food sensitivities.

4. Other, less common factors that might cause or contribute to wetting are the following:

   • Disorders such as polyuria, diabetes, and sickle cell disease
   • Urine infections
   • ADHD
   • Apnea and other sleep disorders
   • Incontinence
   • Stress and reinforcement

In the next chapter, we will consider the psychological effects and complications of bedwetting. You will learn what you can do to encourage your child to keep a positive outlook while he or she tries to get to dry.

Questions and Answers

Q: *My seven-year-old son uses an inhaler for his asthma, especially in the spring and summer. Would his wetting have anything to do with the medication he's on?*

A: Treatments for asthma that involve the use of the drug theophylline (or its congeners), especially if taken orally, can induce bladder symptoms of frequency, urgency, and wetting. However, most asthma treatments nowadays try to avoid medications that are taken orally with the intention of being absorbed by the gastrointestinal tract. Instead, treatments may be taken orally as an aerosol, for local absorption by the lungs. So it is unlikely that contemporary asthma medications are hindering wetting treatment.

On the other hand, Ditropan, a medication we use to treat enuresis (see "Oxybutynin," page 130), is recognized as *possibly* contributing to bronchospasm (asthma). We have not noted this experience in our practice, however.

Q: *My daughter was diagnosed recently with sleep apnea. If we treat her for this condition, is her wetting likely to stop?*

A: Once your child is treated for sleep apnea, if the wetting does not resolve by itself, then you will find it likely to respond to the treatments in this book. If the apnea goes untreated, you may find that the treatment for wetting will not be as effective.

CHAPTER 3

Psychological Issues Associated with Wetting

FOR YEARS, millions of parents have heard the same advice: "Don't worry, your child will outgrow bedwetting." But why should parents accept such an answer, when "outgrowing it" is never offered as a solution for other childhood medical conditions? Sure, most children do eventually "outgrow" wetting, but we don't ignore or accept tooth decay in toddlers because a new set of teeth will come in later. We don't ignore or accept childhood obesity because we hope the child will slim down in adolescence. We don't ignore or accept facial acne in teenagers because it usually disappears in young adulthood.

We encourage good dental hygiene in our toddlers, to protect them against the effects of tooth decay and the poor self-image associated with rotten teeth. We treat obese children with a healthy diet and exercise to prevent obesity in adulthood, which is associated with medical illness, poor self-image, and discrimination. We treat acne with creams and medications to prevent facial scars and to minimize harm to the teen's self-image. Likewise, we should treat wetting problems to protect a child's self-esteem, to promote healthy social development, and to enhance the family's well-being—to say nothing about the expense and labor saved by lightening the laundry load.

In this chapter, we consider the possible psychological causes and effects of wetting conditions. We will show you how children and adults deal with the wetting, both negatively and positively. And we will show you how to maintain a loving and supportive environment while your child is trying to get to dry. But first, we need to expose the truth behind several destructive myths and correct some misconceptions about wetting, people who wet, and their families.

Myths, Misconceptions, and Reality

MYTH: Bedwetters are psychologically disturbed. In earlier times, the collective wisdom of the medical and psychiatric professions had it that enuresis was the manifestation of some underlying unconscious conflict the child was experiencing. In other words, bedwetters were considered psychologically disturbed. From a psychiatric or psychological perspective, children wet because they felt angry or guilty. Doctors believed that if you removed the symptom (wetting) without treating the "real" problem (the underlying unconscious conflict), that conflict would surface in the form of another symptom or behavioral problem.

REALITY: Children who bedwet are no more likely to show psychological disturbance than their nonwetting peers. So it is not surprising that researchers have found that treating enuresis with traditional play therapy, aimed at identifying underlying conflicts, is not very helpful in remitting the wetting. Furthermore, children who have stopped wetting actually feel better about themselves and display no substitute symptoms. If wetting were the symptom of an underlying psychological problem, then after wetting stopped, children would be expected to display another behavioral or emotional problem in its place. Instead, children who have stopped wetting show increased self-esteem.

These notions apply to the majority of children who wet. Nevertheless, a very small minority of children with daytime wetting do wet in an angry, manipulative way—urinating right in front of their parents or in some obvious place (such as on the kitchen floor or in the parents' closet), where the parent is bound to discover the wetting. For these children, wetting is usually a symptom of their psychological problems. Children who engage in such behaviors certainly need a professional evaluation.

Enuretic children show no higher incidence of psychological problems than their friends who do not wet. However, psychological issues do interact with diseases and conditions such as bedwetting. As we will discuss later in this chapter, our emotional well-being influences not only our vulnerability to wetting problems but also our progress toward dryness.

MYTH: Bedwetters are "immature." During toilet training, parents praise and encourage their child when he uses the potty: "You're such a big kid!" If the child does not achieve total bladder control when expected, parents or others may scold him: "You're still a baby." The wet child—and his siblings and friends—gets the pejorative message that something is wrong with him. His parents, who naturally would like to take pride in how grown-up their child is becoming, may act disappointed or embarrassed. In our competitive society, when children do not

PARENTAL MISCONCEPTIONS

According to a recent survey conducted by *USA Today:*

- Eighty percent of parents in the United States do not recognize bedwetting as a medical condition.
- Most parents view bedwetting as a behavioral quirk.
- Twenty percent of parents think that their child wets because he or she is just lazy.
- Twenty percent of parents punish their children for wetting.
- Bedwetting affects five to seven million children in the United States at any one time.

achieve developmental milestones (such as walking, talking, or controlling their bladder) as quickly as their parents expect, their parents may feel like failures or worry that the child is "slow" or developmentally delayed. By the time a child who wets enters preschool or grade school, she may feel immature compared to her peers because she still wets.

REALITY: There is no "normal" age for all children to be dry. Some children are fully toilet trained by three years old, and the majority of children have acceptable bladder control by age five, but remember: the age at which children achieve total bladder control varies according to each individual; the majority of children who wet are not developmentally delayed. On the other hand, a minority of children who wet have been diagnosed by their pediatrician or psychologist as "mentally retarded." Such children not only show a delay in toilet training and attaining dryness but also display significant delays in acquiring other skills as well as intellectual deficits (i.e., IQs of less than 70). Most such children, however, can get to dry, especially if they follow the suggestions in this book.

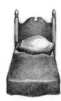

VOICES OF REASON

Throughout history enuretic children have been suspected of laziness and punished relentlessly. According to Dr. Lucille Barash Glicklich, in her article "An Historical Account of Enuresis," an early voice of reason appeared in 1844, when Dr. Samuel Adams stated that he was unwilling to admit that a child ever deliberately wet himself. In what appeared to be an attempt to stir the medical profession to action, he observed, "None of the brute creation will lie in their own urine if they are not tied or penned; why then do we attribute this practice in the rational being to laziness? Simply because some are not able, by careless and superficial examination to find cause . . . they too often condemn the helpless child to daily floggings."

Five decades later, Holt's classic *Textbook of Pediatrics* (1897) declared that "punishments, whether corporal or otherwise, do no good and in most cases are absolutely harmful." Unfortunately, even today children are often blamed, ridiculed, and punished for wetting.

MYTH: Bedwetters are just too lazy to get out of bed and use the toilet. Older children who wet may be accused of being lazy or unwilling to control a simple bodily function. Their parents may ask, "Can't you even get out of bed for a few minutes to pee at night?"

REALITY: Think about it—who would choose to sleep in a cold, wet bed? Children who wet often sleep so deeply that they don't feel, or sense, the urge to urinate. Others may sense the need to void but "dream" that they are at the toilet, and start to urinate not realizing that they are still in bed. As we will see in Chapter 5, the use of an enuresis alarm can help awaken a child who needs to urinate.

MYTH: All children outgrow enuresis. As we have seen, many doctors offer the hopeful advice that parents should just bear

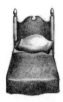

BY THE NUMBERS

Each year about 15 percent of the children who bedwet spontaneously stop wetting; statistically, between 2 and 5 percent of children between ages 12 and 15 continue to wet the bed regularly. So, on average, in a ninth-grade class of 100 students, about three students may continue to wet the bed on a regular basis.

with a wetting problem until the child outgrows it. We hear practically nothing about young and middle-aged adults who wet (as distinct from incontinent seniors).

REALITY: In fact, 1 to 3 percent of the adult population (excluding people who are elderly or neurologically impaired) have enuresis. There is anecdotal evidence that for some adults, stresses they experience (such as college exams, personal relationships, alcohol use, and service in the armed forces) are associated with a reappearance of a childhood wetting problem. Some people with this condition are so secretive and ashamed that they manage to hide the problem—with great difficulty—even from their spouses. So there is nothing magical about the aging process that cures wetting.

MYTH: Children wet because they come from dysfunctional families. It's a notion as old as the problem itself: wetting is the family's fault. If a child wets, she must be showing the effects of living in an unhappy home.

REALITY: Psychopathology probably occurs no more often in families with children who wet than it does in other families. Research shows that most wetting is not caused by psychological problems alone, although for some children who have been dry previously, family stress is associated with the onset of wetting. In addition, when children wet, their family's difficulties may prevent them from outgrowing or overcoming the problem.

For example, it is common for two parents who are already in conflict over other issues to use the child's wetting as another battleground, especially if they disagree about the causes and treatment of the wetting. To spite the other parent, one parent might intentionally undermine the treatment program—for example, by allowing the child to go to bed without putting on the enuresis alarm. Other, less mundane behaviors may also occur. In one case, we treated a child for bedwetting with no success until the mother finally admitted that the father was psychotic. He would inexplicably go into the child's room at night and rip the enuresis alarm out of the child's underwear. It's no wonder that she wasn't making progress. When families can begin to recognize and work around the obstacles they themselves place on the path to dryness, children are much more likely to benefit from treatment.

MYTH: Parents of children with wetting problems have failed to raise their children adequately. Some parents come to us feeling ashamed that they have somehow failed, despite their best efforts, to toilet-train their children. At times their feelings have arisen because a spouse or other family member has blamed the parent for the child's wetting. These parents hear recriminations such as, "If only you did a better job . . . William wouldn't have this problem."
REALITY: Inadequate parenting rarely causes wetting problems. As we have explained, wetting problems have many causes. Unfortunately, parents feel a great deal of unnecessary guilt because of their children's wetting.

How Children React to Their Wetting Problems

By age six, most children who wet realize that they are in the minority among their peers. By age seven, most have become certain that there are no other children in the world their age who still wet—and they do all they can to protect their secret. They become masters at hiding the problem from friends and, to some degree, family. Young and older children might try to hide their soiled bedclothes. Older children might go so far as to secretly wash their own sheets and pajamas. Children who wet during the day sometimes attempt to prepare for any future "accidents" by putting on dark pants and very long T-shirts when they get dressed in the morning. Some children will flatly deny being wet, even when their pants are obviously soaked. They will tell their parents and the doctors, "I don't know why we're doing this treatment. I don't have a problem."

Each child is an individual, and each responds differently to his or her wetting problem. Some appear indifferent, some depressed. All too often, they have just given up hope of getting dry, and may astound you with their seeming acceptance of the condition. To help you recognize your own child's reaction, here are a few common responses that children have to wetting.

"I HAVE TO KEEP IT A SECRET"

Children and grown-ups alike can be cruel. Whether intending to injure or not, people who make jokes or hurtful comments about a child's wetting problem can do serious damage. Children who feel belittled and humiliated about their wetting—by even the slightest hint of disapproval from their parents, siblings, or peers—are more likely to feel bad about themselves as persons. Likewise, when other people shun a child because of his wetting problem, the resulting feelings of isolation can have a whole host of other psychological effects.

To avoid being labeled a bedwetter, children keep their condition a secret. Long-term wetting may eventually impair a child's self-esteem and social development. Because most people—

young and old alike—are uninformed about the basic causes of enuresis, they tend to think and talk about the problem as if wetting is the child's fault. Children who take this finger-pointing to heart may feel shamed and different from their peers and siblings; they feel defective or immature. A child who wets usually feels as though she must be the only child in the world who wets, and she worries that her friends will not like her or will tease her if they find out about the wetting. Children who wet their pants during the day have an especially difficult time: not only is their problem in plain view for all to see and smell, they are also often subjected to teasing and other forms of cruelty by their classmates and neighbors.

Parents may share their child's desire for secrecy because they may know no other families who are struggling with wetting problems. Many parents try to hide a wetting problem in an effort to protect their child from teasing.

"I CAN'T GO ALONG"

Long-term wetting can impair a child's social development because of such secret-keeping. Children live in fear that their secret will come out, so they avoid putting themselves in situations where their wetting might be detected. They refrain from activities that require sleeping away from home, thus missing out on slumber parties, overnight camps, and other events that could build their independence and self-esteem. This abstention from activities, by itself, can make children feel different from their peers and socially isolated.

"I HAVE TO LIE"

To keep their wetting a secret, children will choose to lie about why they cannot join their peers in social activities. Parents may

OUT OF THE CLOSET

People suffering from all types of medical problems—along with their loved ones—have become more aware of the importance of "coming out of the closet." For example, the "insanity" label no longer sticks to those who experience seizures, in part because of the efforts of people who talked openly about their condition. Everyone now recognizes seizure disorders as neurological problems. Similarly, many celebrities as well as medical authorities in the field of attention deficit hyperactivity disorder (ADHD) have acknowledged having this condition. ADHD is now losing its stigma and has standing as a problem with a medical basis. And when it comes to HIV, the virus that causes AIDS, more and more victims and their families have stepped forward. When celebrities such as Magic Johnson talk openly and honestly about their illness, they earn the respect of many people and help lift the burden of shame from their fellow victims. Children who wet have benefited from Northwestern University football coach Gary Barnett's public admission of his own bedwetting as a youth (see "A Role Model," page 67). If other prominent people would also come forward, it would help more children who wet and their families to overcome the shame and secrecy that accompany wetting.

even encourage a child to make up an excuse, or they may lie themselves in an effort to protect the child. Although their motivation may be reasonable, in trying to protect the child the parents reinforce the idea that wetting is shameful. Well-meaning parents may even resort to teaching the child to lie about his wetting, thus sending the message that personal problems must be denied to others. Such secrecy only perpetuates the child's sense of shame, and it conveys the idea that one cannot seek support from others when dealing with problems. Children demeaned by their parents may respond by resorting to lying about their wetting and may hide their wet underwear after they have seen how angry or disappointed their parents become over an episode of wetting.

When children feel that they have to hide their wetting from their parents, a problem greater than the wetting has developed. It then becomes essential to work with your child, along with your doctor, to regain the trust that has been lost. Parents need to let their children know that trust and honesty in their relationship are more important than dryness. In our experience, when parents promise they will not yell at or punish a child for wetting, they usually can get a commitment from the child to be honest. If lying becomes a continuing problem, the family should seek the help of a pediatric mental health professional.

"LEAVE ME ALONE"

Oftentimes well-meaning parents and family members, in their efforts to help an enuretic child, resort to nagging the child to "try harder" to stay dry. Other family members, such as grandparents, may question the child at family get-togethers about how the child is progressing toward dryness. In these situations, children often experience great pressure from the family and, when they have not yet become dry, feel as if they are always disappointing others. Such children may think, "The only thing people care about is whether I'm dry." Such children may resort to avoiding certain family members or lash out in anger: "Leave me alone! Stop bugging me about it!"

"I DON'T CARE"

Although some children seem indifferent to their condition, be assured that their wetting affects them very deeply. Most apparently unconcerned children have likely come to believe that

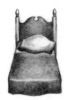

A LESSON IN CARING

Maurice Sendak's *Pierre* is one book you may want to share with very young children who claim not to care about their wetting. Every time his weary mother and father ask him what he wants, the apathetic title character in this classic picture book simply responds, "I don't care." After a hungry lion comes to his home and swallows him whole, with no protest from Pierre, his parents insist that the lion let him out. Eventually, Pierre's parents' perseverance in getting him back helps him see the value of having a loving family.

It's an important message to send to your young one: Just as Pierre's parents kept trying to help him even though he wasn't complaining about being inside the lion's belly, your child needs to know that you will help her find a solution to her wetting problem, even when she has trouble showing how much it bothers her.

nothing can be done for them, so they have given up. If they defensively deny that wetting bothers them, it's because the problem is so painful and humiliating for them. Under such a casual attitude there can hide a scared, ashamed child.

"I'M NOT GOING TO DO IT"

Sometimes when children have been unsuccessful at previous attempts to become dry, they become "oppositional"—that is, uncooperative and contrary—about trying a new treatment approach or seeing a new doctor, or both. Such children lack confidence in anyone's ability to help them with their wetting problem. For some children, having to work on this problem yet another time and having to talk to yet another stranger can be humiliating and dejecting. They come to feel bad about themselves not only because of their wetting problem, but also because of their failure in previous treatment efforts. These children may reject another treatment or another doctor not because they want to keep wetting but because they are afraid to risk another failure.

If they have been humiliated due to their wetting, some children resist participating in treatment because they fear being blamed again, or they feel that it is too embarrassing or painful to discuss. To enlist a child's cooperation and participation in a treatment, parents, health-care providers, and others involved must demonstrate their patience, understanding, and support. This involves normalizing the wetting and addressing it in a neutral manner, not in a blaming or destructive way. Children who are oppositional to treatment can often overcome their resistance with more reinforcers. (For details, see "Additional Reinforcers," page 165, and "Oppositional Behavior," page 195.)

Under some circumstances—for example, when a child is resistant even to try to comply with the treatment program—we recommend making a privilege contingent on compliance. Therefore, if the child wants to watch a video, she has to agree to wear the urine alarm that night and be cooperative. But we present it not in a threatening manner ("If you don't wear your alarm, you're not watching that video!") but in a positive one ("If you want to watch your video tomorrow, you need to wear your alarm when you go to bed tonight").

"I'M ASHAMED OF MYSELF"

The most harmful comments and behaviors can come from the child's own parents: calling their child absent-minded or irresponsible, and then threatening or punishing him when he doesn't control his accidents. (Many parents simply don't realize that their child can't control himself.) People who were belittled for the same problem themselves when they were children may instinctively demean their own child who wets. Parents who use shame can help erode a child's self-esteem, which can result in the child developing behavioral and emotional problems and can undermine the child's efforts to get to dry.

"I KNOW THIS WETTING PROBLEM ISN'T MY FAULT"

Fortunately, many children have supportive families who have accepted their child's wetting problem for what it is: a condition out of their child's direct control. When families don't make a big issue out of wetting, their children may even choose to share their wetting problem with their best friends and their extended family. They also tend to be more enthusiastic about working out ways to join in on sleepovers and other social activities.

IN SUMMARY, as opposed to psychological problems causing wetting, *wetting can cause* low self-esteem, social isolation, missed socialization opportunities, teasing by siblings and peers, conflict between children and parents, and conflict between parents.

Parents, Families, and Bedwetting

Many families choose to deal with a child's wetting by ignoring the situation. They simply deny that there is a problem because they secretly believe that the situation is hopeless. In one recent survey of families of bedwetters, 60 percent of the respondents considered the problem to be incurable.

You can't afford to ignore your child's wetting. If your child is to achieve dryness, she'll need support and positive reinforcement from everyone around her, but the number one supporter must be you, her parent. Your child expects a lot of you. She expects you to have all the answers—or at least to find them. She knows that if anyone will help her get through this uncomfortable time, you will. As we emphasize throughout this book, the task ahead requires patience, consistency, and reassurance.

PARENTS

There are two critical roles for parents to play: nurturer and coach. Much of what needs to be done to treat enuresis falls to your child to do herself, but she will need your understanding, encouragement, and, at times, firm insistence if she is to attain her dream of dry nights and dry clothes. This is not the time to chastise, scold, or punish, no matter how frustrated you become. Keep in mind that your child is frustrated, too. Dr. Stanford Friedman, an expert in the effects of corporal punishment on children, says that parents who use corporal punishment to address their child's bedwetting problem do so out of frustration with not being able to solve the problem in any other way. Parents who use this severe treatment are in the minority, and we hope that, as successful methods of treating enuresis become more widely known, all parents will refrain from resorting to harsh punishment when dealing with their wet children.

Whatever treatments you decide to use, it is important that parents be unified in their support of the program. Today a child may live with one or two parents—biological, foster, or adoptive—in one or two households, as well as with stepparents or grandparents. For the sake of the child, all adults involved as parental figures must be informed and supportive of the chosen treatment plan. When parents openly disagree about a treatment plan, the child may get inconsistent messages about the importance of her compliance with the program, and she can also lose confidence in the treatment. Children may thwart otherwise good efforts by using their parents' disagreement over this issue to play one against the other. Because the child's ability to comply with the prescribed treatment plan is the essence of its success, parents must present an encouraging attitude and united front.

Parents, as well, need support during treatment. They can help each other through the fatigue of interrupted sleep and the frustration of slow or little progress. Parents often find it helpful to take turns getting up with the child during the night, particularly when an alarm is being used.

SIBLINGS

Brothers and sisters can be just as cruel and hurtful to a wet child as the kids at school. To counteract some siblings' tendencies to make insulting comments, be sure to clearly explain your child's wetting problem, and the treatment program you have chosen, to everyone in the immediate family. There is no point in trying to keep the wetting a secret within the family; trying to do so will only reinforce the idea that wetting is shameful. Give brothers and sisters ample opportunity to ask you questions about the wetting and its causes, and ask them to tell you about their own feelings regarding their sibling's problem.

It is also important to encourage your children to help their enuretic sibling deal with individual wetting episodes in a dignified manner. In the case of daytime wetting, rather than laugh and make fun of him, brothers or sisters should either say nothing or acknowledge the "accident" and offer to, say, hold the game, pause the movie, or entertain their friends until the child returns in dry clothes. If the child wets in the presence of other children who notice, his brother or sister can explain, "It's not his fault. He can't help it. But my mom and dad are helping him get over it."

Nevertheless, siblings, who may be resentful because the child with enuresis has gotten so much parental attention, should not be given the message that it is their job to take care of their enuretic sibling; it is the parents' job. Siblings, however, should be willing to stop play while the enuretic child goes to the bathroom. In the case of nighttime wetting, if a sibling is awakened in the middle of the night, one parent should reassure the brother or sister that everything is fine, and help him or her get back to sleep, if necessary.

OUTSIDE THE IMMEDIATE FAMILY

Other people with whom the child has regular contact when wetting might happen need to know about the child's problem and the steps that you and the child are taking to address it. Aunts, uncles, grandparents, and other family members need to learn the basics of wetting and what the treatment program involves. Others who may need to be informed are sitters, au pairs, teachers, and coaches. Treatment programs, particularly for day wetting, often require the assistance of school or day-care personnel to help the child become dry. If the child is willing to go to sleepovers, the host of the sleepover will need guidance as to how to prevent or deal with wetting.

Not everyone will react to your child's wetting in an encouraging manner. It is impossible to protect your child from every situation. When she is confronted with harmful comments or behavior, you should explain to your child that some people do not know the proper way to respond to her wetting.

Summary

Once you recognize the potential psychological and emotional harm that your child may suffer due to a wetting problem, you can begin to play your part in minimizing the damage. To reinforce your child's ability to get to dry, follow this list of suggestions, some of which we have already discussed in this chapter:

DON'TS

- Don't *under any circumstances* make your child feel ashamed of wetting. Shaming has no place in any successful treatment of wetting. Shame and humiliation can cause serious damage to a child's self-esteem and can hurt your relationship with your child.
- Don't get so frustrated and angry that you say or do something hurtful to your child—and it's understandable that you might. So, please, remove yourself to another room of the house until you have calmed down. Unfortunately, many adults who were enuretic as children still recall the terrible humiliation they experienced at the hands of their parents and siblings.
- Don't punish your child for wetting. Instead, try taking a positive approach in which your child can earn praise and rewards for compliance and for attaining dryness.

DO'S

- Acknowledge the involuntary nature of your child's wetting problem. Explain the physiology of bedwetting to your child, using the diagrams and descriptions in Chapter 1, if you need to. Tell your child that you understand that he cannot keep himself from wetting, and that you are willing to help. If enuresis runs in the family, tell your child.
- Shield your child from teasing. Make sure that siblings and other relatives are not labeling or insulting your child. If you hear anyone—whether a neighborhood kid or an unenlightened teacher—taunt or harass your child about her problem, make it clear that you will not tolerate hurtful comments or

behavior. Children with enuresis or incontinence similarly should not be permitted to tease their siblings with hurtful comments regarding their own problems (such as being over-weight or having a tic). If siblings humiliate an enuretic child, they should lose an important privilege and/or get an immedi-ate timeout. Try to explain to the teaser the true nature of bedwetting: it's a medical problem. And make sure you ex-plain to your child that some people do not know the proper way to respond to her wetting, but that's their problem, not hers.

- Resolve to protect your child from conflicts between you and your spouse over the child's wetting problem. On top of han-dling her own social difficulties, a child who feels responsible for her parents' arguments can sink under a burden of guilt and a negative self-image.

- If your child wishes, develop ways to handle sleepovers and other overnight trips so that your child's peers can begin to understand that wetting need not be shameful. One family suggested that at sleepovers, every guest should wear a card-board "decoy" enuresis alarm, just like the host child's real one. That way, they all could experience their friend's pro-gram together. This approach may be too progressive for many families, but it serves as a reminder that the road to further acceptance of bedwetting as a medical problem begins with small, courageous steps.

- Be consistent in following through with any attempted treat-ment program. If you are inconsistent, the program will likely be ineffective and set up the child for failure. Avoid blaming the child, and instead encourage him to do what needs to be done to gain control (namely, take responsibility) of the situation.

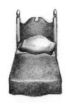

A ROLE MODEL

In his recent autobiography, *High Hopes,* Northwestern University football coach Gary Barnett revealed his own childhood bedwetting. He described the distress he felt from being labeled a bedwetter: having to sleep on plastic sheets, being barred from spending the night at a friend's house, and hearing his father threaten to hang Gary's dirty linen out the window and throw his soiled mattress on the front lawn. According to Gary, his bedwetting continued into his sophomore year in high school; it "mercifully" stopped the night before his first high school football game. "I never did find out why it happened," he told us. "I survived it, but I was pretty fragile for a long time." If more people in the public eye would acknowledge having had a wetting problem, we might see a different response from our neighbors and friends.

Questions and Answers

Q: *I'll be working with kids—ages five to fifteen, boys and girls—at the YMCA camp this summer. How should I deal with younger kids who wet, as opposed to ten-year-olds or teens? What about the differences between boys and girls in how they react when they wet?*

A: All camps should request information on registration forms and on medical history forms from parents about any behavioral and/or medical problems the child has. Some camp forms specifically inquire about bedwetting. Children should not bring their enuresis alarms to camp. (We discuss enuresis alarms in Chapter 5.) The camp director and counselor should plan to talk to the parents of enuretic children before camp begins about how best to handle the wetting. Therefore, an individualized response can be prepared for a child based on his situation and feelings.

Some children may wish to keep their wetting a secret; others may feel relieved not to have to hide their problem. If the child wants to keep wetting a secret, the counselors should talk to the child on the first day of camp and make a plan of how a wet bed can be changed without drawing attention to the problem. Particularly if it is the child's choice to keep the bedwetting a secret, the camper needs to be given the opportunity to return to the cabin in the morning to change her bed in private. Children who do not want to keep their wetting a secret may also appreciate the counselor's explaining to the campers in the cabin that the child's wetting is due to a medical problem over which the child has no control. Any teasing by other campers should be prohibited.

Although older children may be more embarrassed by wetting problems than younger children, all children with wetting should be treated with respect. We do not know if there is a difference in the way in which boys and girls react to their wetting, although in our experience there does not seem to be any difference. The counselors can remind all children to use the bathroom before bed, so as not to single out the enuretic child. At some overnight camps, counselors wake the child with a wetting problem and take him to the bathroom before they go to sleep.

Parents of children who have a daytime wetting problem must also make arrangements with camp personnel regarding the best way to handle accidents. These children can be on a timed voiding program—that is, make scheduled trips to the bathroom—if the parents and health-care professional agree. (We discuss timed voiding in Chapter 6.) Children with diurnal enuresis need to have a change of clothes nearby in case it is needed.

Q: *How do I know when to get psychological counseling for my child? How can I tell whether he's clinically depressed or just a little down about his wetting?*

A: You should seek psychological counseling for your child if your child's problems interfere with his functioning in one or more areas (such as academic performance, social functioning, relationships with family members, self-care, and so on) and/or if they cause significant distress.

Major depression, often referred to as clinical depression, is when a child or adolescent is nearly always depressed or very irritable and/or displays a loss of interest or pleasure for at least a two-week period, and the depression impairs functioning and causes distress. Major depression is not usually caused by a minor stress, and the child does not have days during this two-week period when he feels happy. To be diagnosed as having a major depression, the child also must display almost daily at least four of the following symptoms: appetite disturbance, sleep problems, restlessness or feeling slowed down, fatigue and lack of energy, feelings of worthlessness, difficulty concentrating or indecisiveness, and recurrent thoughts of death or suicidal ideation.

There is no indication that enuresis causes depression, unlike, say, hypothyroidism (a disease of the thyroid gland), which causes clinical depressive symptoms. It is more likely that a child may be "down" about her wetting because it prevents her from engaging in certain activities or has resulted in teasing and loss of self-esteem. These "down" periods are short-lived, rarely lasting more than a couple of hours. In our experience, parents who are supportive of their enuretic children and avoid blaming or humiliating them are likely to have children who can cope with this problem. Additionally, the children we have seen in our clinic who have been clinically depressed do not suffer this disorder because of their wetting problem.

Q: *I'm confused about the whole privacy issue. First you say that children need to be protected from teasing, but then you say that keeping secrets is unhealthy? Can you elaborate?*

A: Enuresis and incontinence are disorders that are medically, not developmentally, based and are not the child's or the parents' "fault." Therefore, a child with a wetting problem needs neither to feel ashamed nor to keep the wetting a secret. Children and their families can educate others about these disorders. Nevertheless, despite such education, some people are either stuck to their old ideas (such as, "that child is just lazy") or are psychologically insensitive or immature. These are people who, despite knowing otherwise, cannot be trusted to be supportive of the child. Therefore, although ideally wetting problems should not have to be kept a secret, families must use their own judgment about who may be told about the wetting. In addition, parents and extended family members must respect the feelings of the child when deciding with whom they will share the information. Obviously, any caretaker of the child needs to be informed so that the caretaker will know how to implement the treatment program and the appropriate way to deal with accidents.

PART TWO

Finding the Solutions

Chapter 4

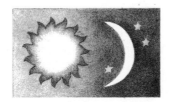

Getting a Clear Picture

MANY FAMILIES still do not realize that the problem of bedwetting is treatable. In fact, it is. In this part of the book, you will learn the details of our treatment plan, the same plan we have used successfully at Children's Memorial Hospital in Chicago for the past decade. Our program maximizes the potential for success because it is *multi-modal*. That is, after we have made a working diagnosis of the causes of wetting in each child, we target the suspected causes with multiple modes, or types, of treatments. The treatments are carried out simultaneously. This diverse set of treatments attacks at the same time what we described earlier as the four most common factors behind wetting problems: (1) deep sleep or failure to arouse from sleep, (2) small bladder capacity, (3) bowel problems, and (4) diet sensitivities.

This program works, but it also takes some work. It requires the family to understand the intent of each individual treatment used. The tasks required are not difficult but may be inconvenient. However, once you and your child experience a few dry nights, your confidence will grow and the work will get easier. Children generally cannot understand why their wetting just won't go away, so it's your job not only to explain each cause and its associated treatment to your child, but also to help keep him on track.

There is a simple reason that we decided to call our program Try for Dry and to name this book *Getting to Dry*. We want to remind children and families alike that the "trying," the ongoing commitment to making a positive change, is fundamental. No treatment program for any medical condition can guarantee 100 percent success, but we believe that if you and your child maintain your optimism and stick to the plan, you will see results and get to dry.

To help you obtain an accurate record of your child's condition, in this chapter we will guide you through the following five steps:

Step 1. Determine what type of wetting problem your child has.
Step 2. Assess whether or not the occurrence of your child's wetting is related to any psychological factors or events.
Step 3. Measure your child's functional bladder capacity.
Step 4. Record how often your child urinates and moves his bowels.
Step 5. Consider whether your child may have any food or beverage sensitivities.

For steps 1 and 2, you will complete the questionnaire that begins on page 76. For steps 3 through 5, you will record your observations in the Three-Day Diary (pages 84–87), which we will explain in detail later in this chapter. Your answers on the questionnaire and the information you record in the diary will serve three purposes: They will (1) help you better understand your child's condition, (2) provide essential information that your doctor will need when he examines your child, and (3) permit you to match the problems that are causing the wetting with the right treatments in Chapters 5 and 6.

In particular, your answers on the following questionnaire will help determine if deep sleep, small bladder size, food sensitivities, or bowel problems occur in your child. If they do, then after consulting your health-care provider, you will likely begin using at least two of the following treatments *simultaneously:* (1) the enuresis alarm (for deep sleep), (2) the medication Ditropan (for the small bladder size), (3) the Happy Bladder Diet (to remove the effects of any food sensitivities), and (4) the bowel program (if defecation is irregular).

MEASURING BLADDER CAPACITY AND URINARY FREQUENCY

Most children who wet have a reduced functional bladder capacity. Although this reduction is not the primary cause of enuresis, it's a good idea to find out what your child's capacity is so that a correct diagnosis can be made. By definition, functional bladder capacity is the largest volume of urine voided *at one time,* as measured during a three-day recording period.

To measure your child's bladder capacity, have him urinate into a container that will allow you to measure the volume of urine. The ideal container is a Specipan, which can be purchased from a medical supply store (see Appendix D). The Specipan fits easily under your home toilet seat so that your child can void normally and comfortably. The Specipan has graduated markings (in ounces) so that you can measure immediately the volume of your child's urine and then dispose of it in the toilet. Depending on the age of your child, you can substitute a plastic bowl, a potty bowl, or other suitable container from which you can pour the contents into a measuring cup. Some people are successful

THE QUESTIONNAIRE

BASIC INFORMATION

Today's Date: _____

Child's Name: _____

Child's Age: _____ years   Child's Gender: ❑ Boy ❑ Girl

Age

1. According to my child's chronological age, his age group is

    ❑ Infant   under 2 years old (and the child does not yet walk)
    ❑ Toddler   2 to 4 years old (or a child under 2 who walks)
    ❑ Youth   5 to 9 years old
    ❑ Preteen   10 to 12 years old
    ❑ Teen   13 to 19 years old
    ❑ Adult   20 or older

Type of Wetting

2. Has your child ever been continent—that is, "dry"—by day and by night for six consecutive months or more? ❑ Yes ❑ No
    *If No, your child has **primary** enuresis.*
    *If Yes, your child has **secondary** enuresis.*

3. Does your child wet while awake? ❑ Yes ❑ No
    *If Yes, the wetting is **diurnal**.*

4. Does your child wet while asleep? ❑ Yes ❑ No
    *If Yes, the wetting is **nocturnal**.*

5. Does your child wet when awake and when asleep? ❑ Yes ❑ No
    *If Yes, the wetting is both **diurnal** and **nocturnal**.*

6. Does your child wet only while giggling or laughing, or perhaps while climbing stairs? ❑ Yes ❑ No
    *If Yes, your child has **giggle wetting**.*

NOTE: These terms can be used in combination. For instance, answering No to question 2 and Yes to question 4 would mean that your child has primary nocturnal enuresis.

7. Has a doctor ever found your child to have a urine infection, or have you ever suspected that your child had a urine infection? ❑ Yes ❑ No
   If Yes, your child's problem with wetting and urine infection may be a sign of incontinence, not enuresis. Make sure to discuss this possibility with your doctor.

Sleep

8. Does your child sleep deeply or heavily? ❑ Yes ❑ No
   If Yes, it is likely that deep sleep is contributing to your child's wetting.

9. Does your child frequently experience problems during sleep, such as night terrors or nightmares, sleepwalking, snoring, or teeth grinding? ❑ Yes ❑ No
   If Yes, your child may have difficulty getting to dry using the treatments in this book. Make sure to discuss these problems with your doctor.

PSYCHOLOGICAL INFORMATION

Stressful Life Events Inventory

Under the categories below, please list all events that have happened in your family over the past twelve months, both positive (such as "parent got a promotion with a raise" or "parents' marriage improved") and negative (such as "sibling became chronically ill" or "grandparent died").

10. Death of a family member or close friend
    a. _____
    b. _____
    c. _____
    d. _____

11. Serious illness in a family member or close friend
    a. _____
    b. _____
    c. _____
    d. _____

12. Marital problems and/or changes in your marriage
    a. _____
    b. _____
    c. _____
    d. _____

13. Emotional or behavioral problems of a family member (including depression, anxiety, ADHD, psychosis, and other disorders), whether or not they have been diagnosed and treated by a mental health professional

    a. _____
    b. _____
    c. _____
    d. _____

14. Birth or adoption in the immediate family

    a. _____
    b. _____
    c. _____
    d. _____

15. Change in finances and/or job

    a. _____
    b. _____
    c. _____
    d. _____

16. School changes and/or problems

    a. _____
    b. _____
    c. _____
    d. _____

17. Drug or alcohol abuse in the immediate family

    a. _____
    b. _____
    c. _____
    d. _____

18. Physical or sexual abuse in the immediate family

    a. _____
    b. _____
    c. _____
    d. _____

Count the items you listed in questions 10 through 18 and write that number below.

    Our family has experienced _____ life events in the past twelve months.

Major changes or events in a child's life may contribute to the onset of wetting in a child who was previously dry. (That is, they may help trigger secondary enuresis.) Such disruptions may also hinder a child's progress in getting dry, whether the child has primary or secondary enuresis.

Relationship Between Parents

19. How would you describe your relationship with your spouse or partner?
   ❑ Mostly happy
   ❑ Both happy and unhappy
   ❑ Mostly unhappy

Parents who are often unhappy in their relationship and engage in conflict may find it difficult to present a positive, united front to the child who wets when implementing the treatment program.

Motivation

Families who succeed in attaining dryness work together, as a team. On the following scales, rate each family member's commitment to this effort, in your opinion:

20. The child who wets is
   1 Not motivated
   2 Slightly motivated
   3 Motivated
   4 Very motivated
   5 Extremely motivated

21. I am
   1 Not motivated
   2 Slightly motivated
   3 Motivated
   4 Very motivated
   5 Extremely motivated

22. My spouse is
   1 Not motivated
   2 Slightly motivated
   3 Motivated
   4 Very motivated
   5 Extremely motivated

23. Overall, other members of the immediate family are
   1 Not motivated
   2 Slightly motivated
   3 Motivated
   4 Very motivated
   5 Extremely motivated

If all family members are motivated to get to dry, then it is likely that the family will succeed in completing this program, and the child's wetting will remit.

However, if the child himself is not motivated, or if you and your spouse do not share the same level of motivation, the treatment plan is unlikely to succeed. If that is the case in your family, you need to work around whatever obstacles are in the way before proceeding (see "Reasons to Consider Delaying Treatment," page 98).

Finally, success does not depend on motivated siblings, but parents should watch for a sibling's attempts to undermine or sabotage the child's treatment plan.

having the child void into a large measuring cup or graduated bowl.

For three days (which do not need to be consecutive), each time your child urinates during daytime hours, write the time of day and the amount of urine in the diary. Also, each time your child wets her clothing during the day, note the time in the appropriate place in the diary. Please also note if she wakes up wet.

Once you have completed this section of the diary, scan the amount column to find the largest volume of urine voided in a single trip to the toilet. This is your child's functional bladder capacity. Now compare that amount to Table 4-1. If your child fits the pattern for primary nocturnal enuresis (that is, deep sleep, small bladder capacity, and no other illnesses), his measurement will fall below the specific range according to the table. On the other hand, if your child's bladder capacity is greater than the norm, be sure to point that out to your doctor, because incontinence, not enuresis, may be a problem.

You should now record your child's functional bladder capacity on the appropriate line in the diary (see page 87).

Urination Frequency and Urgency

Children, on average, urinate six times per day. A child has a problem with urination frequency if he or she urinates fewer than four times a day (too infrequent) or more than nine times a day (too frequent). Also, the child's urination should not routinely be urgent.

Frequency. Using the urination times you have recorded in the diary, compare your child's urination frequency to the average frequency. Most children urinate right after they get up in the morning, and then one or two times in each of the following

TIPS FOR USING THE DIARY

- While keeping the diary, *do not prompt your child to void.* Let him urinate according to his own body cues. We are trying to determine the maximum amount of urine that the child's bladder can empty, which most of the time is also the maximum amount the child can hold when he has the urge to "go." If you suggest that he empty his bladder before it is full, this may result in an underestimation of the functional bladder capacity.
- Even if your child is responsible enough to measure his own urine and record the time of voiding, please make sure that you *personally* supervise this activity. After all, the use of prescription medication may depend on the information in the diary. Let's be sure that it is as accurate as possible.
- If it seems that your child is intrigued by the diary and goes to the toilet much more often than usual for him, just wait until the "fascination" phase is over. Then go ahead and start your measurements.
- There is no need for you to measure the volume of urine voided during wetting episodes. We realize that it is impractical to do so.

intervals: 8:00 A.M. to noon, noon to 4:00 P.M., and 4:00 P.M. to bedtime. In the appropriate place in the diary, note the frequency of your child's urination and whether it is less than average, average, or more than average.

Urgency. Also, note in the diary whether or not your child often shows an urgent need to void. Naturally, measuring a child's urinary urgency is very subjective, but if her need is so great that you often have to stop at public restrooms on car trips, at malls, and in other situations, your child may have urinary urgency.

TABLE 4-1. Predicted Normal Functional Bladder Capacity

Age (years)	Predicted Normal Range (ounces)	Average (ounces)
5	5–9	7
6	6–10	8
7	7–11	9
8	8–12	10
9	9–13	11
10	10–14	12
11 +	11–15	13

OBSERVING BOWEL FREQUENCY

Because of the close relationship between good bladder control and bowel regularity, it is important that your child have regular daily bowel movements. In children who wet, constipation could "irritate" the bladder and complicate their ability to get to dry. In order to determine whether or not your child is constipated, record in the diary every time your child moves his bowels during the three-day period. Then answer the following detailed questions in the diary regarding your child's stooling:

- Do you think your child is constipated?
- Does your child have a bowel movement every day?
- How often does your child have a bowel movement?
- Are your child's bowel movements usually painful for him?
- Does your child stain his underpants with stool?
- What consistency, on average, are the stools: hard, normal, or loose?
- What size, on average, are the stools: small, medium, or large?
- Does your child complain frequently about stomach pain?

If your child does not have a daily bowel movement, has pain upon defecation, has soiling of the underpants (e.g., encopresis), or hard consistency of stool, then he shows "irregular bowels." This irregularity will need to be addressed before starting the Try for Dry program (see "Improving Bowel Health," page 147). When you are recording information about bowel movements, make sure you inspect the toilet for evidence of defecation. Though most younger children will yield their privacy about such matters, many older children are reluctant to have someone observe their bowel movements. Reassure your child that this breach of his privacy will only last a few days and that his chances of getting dry will be much better if the information about his bowel movements is accurate. We have found that many parents do not recognize their child's constipation problem until they carefully observe the child's toileting habits over a few days.

FOOD SENSITIVITIES

Over the three days that you are recording your child's urination and defecation (preferably the same three days during which you are recording the urine and bowel patterns), you should note what foods your child is eating, what fluids she is drinking, the amounts of foods and fluids, and the times at which they are consumed. If she has a sandwich for lunch, be specific: Was it ham and cheese or peanut butter and jelly? Did the pizza have pepperoni and mushrooms, or was it plain cheese? Was the juice she drank 25 percent apple or 100 percent orange?

In Chapter 6, we will lead you through the steps of administering the Happy Bladder Diet to your child, in an effort to isolate specific problem foods. In the meantime, you should plan to share this information about your child's diet with your doctor. The more detailed your diary is, the more accurate the conclusions that you and your doctor will be able to reach.

THE THREE-DAY DIARY

day one

URINATION

Time	Amt. of Urine Voided (oz.)	Are Clothes Wet or Dry?
		❏ wet ❏ dry
	✱	❏ wet ❏ dry
		❏ wet ❏ dry
		❏ wet ❏ dry
		❏ wet ❏ dry
		❏ wet ❏ dry
		❏ wet ❏ dry
		❏ wet ❏ dry
		❏ wet ❏ dry

My child woke up ❏ wet   ❏ dry.

BOWEL ELIMINATION

My child had a bowel movement today: ❏ Yes ❏ No
If Yes, the time was _____ .

    The movement was painful for my child: ❏ Yes ❏ No
    My child's underpants were stained with stool: ❏ Yes ❏ No
    The consistency of the stool was ❏ hard ❏ normal ❏ loose.
    The size of the stool was ❏ small ❏ medium ❏ large.

FOOD AND BEVERAGES

Time	Food/Bev. Consumed	Amount

URINATION

Time	Amt. of Urine Voided (oz.)	Are Clothes Wet or Dry?
		❏ wet ❏ dry
		❏ wet ❏ dry
		❏ wet ❏ dry
		❏ wet ❏ dry
		❏ wet ❏ dry
		❏ wet ❏ dry
		❏ wet ❏ dry
		❏ wet ❏ dry
		❏ wet ❏ dry
		❏ wet ❏ dry

My child woke up ❏ wet ❏ dry.

BOWEL ELIMINATION

My child had a bowel movement today: ❏ Yes ❏ No
If Yes, the time was _____ .

The movement was painful for my child: ❏ Yes ❏ No
My child's underpants were stained with stool: ❏ Yes ❏ No
The consistency of the stool was ❏ hard ❏ normal ❏ loose.
The size of the stool was ❏ small ❏ medium ❏ large.

FOOD AND BEVERAGES

Time	Food/Bev. Consumed	Amount

URINATION

Time	Amt. of Urine Voided (oz.)	Are Clothes Wet or Dry?
		❑ wet ❑ dry
		❑ wet ❑ dry
		❑ wet ❑ dry
		❑ wet ❑ dry
		❑ wet ❑ dry
		❑ wet ❑ dry
		❑ wet ❑ dry
		❑ wet ❑ dry
		❑ wet ❑ dry
		❑ wet ❑ dry

My child woke up ❑ wet   ❑ dry.

BOWEL ELIMINATION

My child had a bowel movement today: ❑ Yes ❑ No
If Yes, the time was _____ .
> The movement was painful for my child: ❑ Yes ❑ No
> My child's underpants were stained with stool: ❑ Yes ❑ No
> The consistency of the stool was ❑ hard ❑ normal ❑ loose.
> The size of the stool was ❑ small ❑ medium ❑ large.

FOOD AND BEVERAGES

Time	Food/Bev. Consumed	Amount

DIARY RESULTS

Urination

By selecting from the diary the largest volume of urine voided at one time over the three-day period, I have determined my child's functional bladder capacity to be _____ ounces.

Compared to the average amount of _____ ounces (from Table 4-1 on page 82) for other children his age who do not wet, my child's functional bladder capacity is
❑ **too low** ❑ **average** ❑ **too high.**

My child's urinary frequency is
❑ **too infrequent** (fewer than 4 times a day)
❑ **normal** (4–9 times a day)
❑ **too frequent** (more than 9 times a day).

In general, my child ❑ **does** ❑ **does not** show urinary urgency.

Bowel Elimination

I believe my child ❑ **has normal defecation** ❑ **is constipated.**
My child ❑ **does** ❑ **does not** have a bowel movement every day.
My child's elimination frequency is _____ days/week.
Pain ❑ **does** ❑ **does not** usually accompany bowel elimination.
In general, there ❑ **is** ❑ **is not** soiling of stool in the underpants.
My child's stool consistency is most often ❑ **hard** ❑ **normal** ❑ **loose.**
The stool size usually appears ❑ **small** ❑ **medium** ❑ **large.**
My child ❑ **does** ❑ **does not** frequently complain of stomach pain.

Food and Beverages

This list is taken from the "Foods to Avoid" section of the Happy Bladder Diet in Chapter 6. Check any of the items that appear in your diary.

❑ Carbonated drinks (Coke, Pepsi, 7-Up, and others)

❑ Caffeinated drinks (coffee, tea, most soda)

❑ Drinks with artificial colors (Kool-Aid, Hawaiian Punch, Hi-C, and others)

❑ Drinks with citric acid (orange juice, lemon juice, grapefruit juice, and others)

❑ Sugary food or candy

❑ Milk and dairy beverages (when consumed after noon)

❑ Pizza with cheese (when consumed after lunch)

❑ Ice cream (after dinner)

❑ Other dairy products (after noon)

❑ Melons (watermelon, cantaloupe, and others)

❑ Vitamin supplements with artificial colors or vitamin C

If you checked one or more boxes, food sensitivities may be contributing to your child's wetting.

Resist the temptation to hide all the candy, soda, and other goodies while you're recording in the diary just because you don't want the doctor to know what your child really eats and drinks. An accurate diary is very helpful in identifying which foods and beverages may make it hard for your child to get to dry.

Visiting Your Doctor

Once you have answered the questionnaire and completed the three-day diary, the next step is the medical examination. Whether a general practitioner, a pediatrician, a nurse practitioner, or other professional, your family health-care provider is the person most familiar with your child's health and history. If you are also consulting a specialist, such as a psychologist, psychiatrist, or other mental health professional for wetting and/or other problems, by all means discuss with her your child's inability to stay dry—and your intention to begin the Try for Dry treatment—but make sure that your child is also evaluated medically for the wetting. This step is absolutely essential because your health-care provider needs to exclude the possibility that incontinence or other health problems may complicate your child's ability to get to dry.

Bring this book with you to the doctor's office, and talk to your doctor about the information you've collected in the questionnaire and the diary. Your doctor will likely already be familiar with some or all of the treatment techniques described in this book, but she may be unfamiliar with our systematic approach.

Your doctor may recommend that you see either of two specialists: a urologist or a nephrologist. Urologists specialize in the treatment of conditions that may require surgery to correct a problem of the urinary tract. Nephrologists specialize in the treatment of conditions associated with medical problems of the kidneys. Seeking advice from either of these specialists is logical and prudent, to check for problems of incontinence. However, keep in mind that, while specialists are overall very knowledgeable in treating children with organic problems associated with incontinence, they may not be aware of the best treatments for enuresis. Most medical schools simply do not yet teach the treatment of enuresis.

Because enuresis is such a common problem, you will find that most health-care practitioners have formulated some answer or method for dealing with it. As we mentioned earlier, your health-care professional might suggest that you do nothing and see if your child "grows out of it." This common tactic works about 15 percent of the time. That is, every year, about 15 percent of the population of enuretic children "win the bladder lottery" and spontaneously stop wetting. You may choose the "wait-and-see" option, but you must consider how long you are willing to wait. If you would like to better your child's odds of attaining dryness soon, then consider the treatment options presented in the following chapters.

THE OFFICE VISIT

Before he examines your child, your doctor will likely ask you some of the same questions you have already answered on our questionnaire. In addition, he is likely to ask at least some of the following questions:

- Does your child exhibit day urgency and frequency? (In other words, could these symptoms be a clue to small functional bladder capacity?)
- Is the wetting associated with abdominal pain? (That is, could the bladder be large and overfull before voiding?)

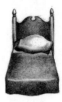

PREPARING YOUR CHILD FOR A WETTING EVALUATION

There are a number of steps you can take to ease any anxiety that your child might feel about her first evaluation for wetting:

- Explain the reason for the visit ahead of time to your child. Make sure she understands that the doctor is someone who can help her stop wetting.
- Reassure your child that this exam will not involve any painful procedures such as blood tests or injections.
- Explain to your child that the doctor will be asking her about her bladder and bowel habits or routines because they might help explain some of her wetting.
- Make sure your child understands the words the doctor will be using. For example, if your family refers to bowel movements as "BMs" and to urination as "tinkling," you should explain what other words the doctor might use. You may also let your doctor know ahead of time which words your family uses for bodily functions, so he or she can use those words when talking to your child.
- If your child seems anxious about the upcoming visit, schedule a "mini-visit" before the actual exam. This can give your child the opportunity to say hello to the doctor and the office staff, perhaps get a sticker or some other prize, and then go home. Just familiarizing a child with the doctor's office often helps her relax about the exam.

Your child's best allies in her struggle to overcome wetting are her parents and her doctor. Help her think of the doctor's examination as another positive step, as a sign of real progress toward getting to dry.

- Has your child ever had a urine infection?
- If the child is a boy: Is his urine stream strong and steady, or weak and variable?
- If the child is a girl: Does she continuously dribble urine?

The Physical Examination

Next, the doctor will examine your child to see whether incontinence may be causing the wetting. To maintain the child's privacy, ask the doctor to place a sheet or towel over the child's lower abdominal area so the child is not completely exposed. Among other things, the doctor will check the following:

- She will examine the genitalia and rectum, and the back and stomach, looking for signs of fecal impaction, constipation, or neurological disorders. For a boy, she will also check the genitals to be sure the urine opening on the penis, called the meatus, is normal. For a girl, she will check the genitalia to be sure the urethra opening is not covered and that there are no extra openings for the passage of urine.
- For either a boy or a girl, the doctor will check the abdomen to see if he can feel a distended bladder or bowel.
- The doctor will examine the back and buttocks to check for external signs of an underlying problem of the spinal nerves to the bladder (such as spina bifida). Such signs include a patch of skin that has too much hair or too much pigmentation, a dimple over the sacrum bone, or one buttock much bigger than the other.
- The doctor will examine the feet and check the knee reflexes (abnormalities here again could signal the presence of an underlying spinal cord problem).
- Finally, the doctor will ask for a urine sample to check for infection, blood, sugar, pH, and urine concentration.

The doctor's physical examination will be quick, and your child should be familiar with some portions of the exam from her routine visits to the pediatrician.

Laboratory Tests

If the doctor suspects incontinence after taking the history and performing the physical exam, he may conduct or order some tests to complete the evaluation. (If he suspects enuresis, he probably will not order the tests.) One test he might perform is an ultrasound—much like the kind expectant mothers undergo. An ultrasound will allow the doctor to determine if the bowel is full and possibly irritating the bladder. It will also show any blockages or possible malformations in the urinary tract. It may show that the bladder is thick walled, that is, "too muscular" and likely to have a spastic emptying pattern. If a child's bladder empties too quickly and urgently, the child can't inhibit the contraction, so she wets.

Rarely, expensive and sophisticated tests of how the bladder works, called urodynamic testing, will be ordered. A urodynamics test will determine whether the muscles involved in emptying the bladder are working together properly and whether the flow of urine is either normal or abnormal, indicating the presence of a blockage of some sort. For boys, the simplest urodynamic test that doctors conduct is observing the boy urinate, noting the quality of the urine stream, especially the force of the stream's flow. For girls, doctors listen to the girl's urine stream as she sits on the toilet: Is there a continuous flow with good force or a "stuttering" stream without good force?

Additional tests might be ordered, such as a voiding cystourethrogram (VCUG), which is a type of bladder X-ray that uses a catheter; an intravenous pyelogram (IVP) (*a.k.a.* excretory urogram), which is a kidney X-ray; or a cystoscopy, which is an examination of the bladder using a miniature telescope.

The Diagnosis: Enuresis or Incontinence?

Based upon all of the information she has gathered, your doctor may suggest one of two diagnoses: enuresis or incontinence. As we explained in Chapter 1, enuresis is a wetting condition in which there is no apparent structural defect in the urinary system. Enuresis, the most likely diagnosis, can be treated—and quite successfully—with the methods that we describe in the following chapters. Incontinence is a wetting condition that results from some abnormality in the urinary tract. Incontinence is usually treated with surgery. (See Appendix C for a brief description of the most common causes of incontinence in children.)

If your doctor suggests that incontinence is the problem, then the child should be examined by a pediatric urologist. Your doctor may suspect that incontinence could be due to a mild disorder (such as meatal stenosis, described in Appendix C) but suggest a simple enuresis treatment to begin with rather than going straight to surgical options. Many times, it is better to try a simple enuresis treatment program—and possibly solve the wetting problem—than to immediately pursue the more complicated surgical remedies for incontinence.

More than likely, however, the diagnosis will be enuresis. If so, you can help your child overcome his wetting problem and get to dry by using the Try for Dry treatments described in this book.

Summary

In this chapter, we have described the information-gathering stage of the process. Answering the questionnaire, keeping the diary, and visiting the doctor all are done with the same goal in mind: to isolate the causes of your child's wetting. In the next chapter, we will help you interpret the facts you have recorded and choose the proper combination of treatments.

Chapter 5

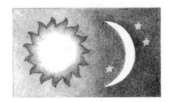

Beginning the Treatments

THE TECHNIQUES that we describe in this chapter have grown out of years of effort by parents, children, medical professionals, and others involved in the treatment of wetting.

One of the reasons that enuresis seems so difficult to cure is that, currently, most other plans attack the problem from only one angle:

". . . Go buy the alarm and give it a try . . ."

". . . Try two puffs of this nose spray . . ."

". . . Don't give any liquids after dinner . . ."

". . . Why don't you think about seeing a psychologist . . ."

In our opinion, most children's enuresis results from more than one factor and requires systematically evaluating and treating all of the known factors and/or symptoms with an organized and comprehensive plan. The current scheme usually offered families is to pick one or possibly two treatment modes and then hope for the best. This hit-or-miss approach sometimes succeeds, but sometimes does not. In addition, since enuresis is known to spontaneously remit, the selected treatment may be credited with an undeserved success.

Our program works because we develop a working diagnosis in an organized way and then pick multiple treatments that are used simultaneously. These diverse treatments attack what we recognize as the most common problems: deep sleep, small bladder capacity, irregular defecation/constipation, and diet.

We are confident that after you match your child's symptoms with the appropriate treatments (see Table 5-1, page 98) and start the program, you will see a significant change within a few weeks. And with the help of the motivational tactics we offer in Chapter 7, the initial successes of the first few nights will continue even after the novelty of the program has worn off.

For your child to maintain his momentum and build permanent dryness habits, however, he needs you to set the stage. To maximize your child's chances of success, please be sure to read and follow these five important suggestions before you proceed:

1. **Make sure the time is right.** If a new baby is due soon, if an illness or divorce is preoccupying the family, or if it is a particularly critical time at work or school, when uninterrupted sleep is a necessity for you or another family member, wait to start this (or any other) program. Rather than begin a new project with such high emotional stakes in a stressful environment, it is much better to delay treatment until the family has adapted to the new routine or other tensions have subsided. For example, if school issues preoccupy your child, hold off until summertime, when school is out and his motivation may be greater. (See "Reasons to Consider Delaying Treatment," page 98, for more details.)

2. **Be sure your child wants to begin the treatments and agrees with your approach.** The effectiveness of any treatment program depends on the child's desire to take responsibility for her own body. If she feels too much parental pressure or has no motivation to become dry, failure is likely.

3. **Do not let your child get overtired.** As we explained in Chapter 2, deep sleep accounts in some measure for almost all night wetting (that is, as primary nocturnal enuresis). After weeks of dry nights, one night of unusually deep sleep can result in a wet bed if the child sleeps too soundly to sense her bladder's signals. If you know your child will be going to bed very tired on a particular night, expect a wet night, but take precautions against wetting. Consider limiting how much fluid he drinks before bedtime, plan to take him to the toilet in the middle of the night when the alarm sounds, and protect his mattress with an absorbent pad and/or plastic mattress cover.

4. **Establish a relaxing bedtime routine, including two trips to the bathroom.** It is important that children empty their bladder completely before bed. A peaceful, orderly bedtime routine will not only make bedtime a happier experience for everyone, but it will also help your child relax enough to void fully. Have your child follow the same sequence of steps every night before sleep, for example: (1) changing into pajamas, (2) visiting the bathroom to brush her teeth and urinate, (3) reading a story with you, (4) getting a goodnight kiss, (5) urinating in the toilet again, and finally (6) lying down for sleep.

5. **Have your child practice getting up at night to go to the bathroom.** Explain to your child that for five nights in a row before the real bedtime, you are going to help her learn to go to the bathroom in the middle of the night. Each night turn

off all the lights (except nightlights) and have your child lie in bed and pretend to be asleep. Then leave the room and wait a minute. Return to her bedroom, gently shake your child, and say, "Come on, honey, time to go to the bathroom." Follow your child and support her as she navigates her way to the bathroom, sits on (or, for a boy, stands at) the toilet and pretends to urinate in the toilet, and then returns to bed. After each practice run, give her lots of affection and praise, and reinforce the idea that she is old enough to get up in the middle of the night by herself when the alarm sounds or when her bladder is full.

Once you feel that you and your child are ready to begin, the next step is to assemble a customized treatment regimen that targets the symptoms you identified in Chapter 4.

Building a Plan

Based on the answers you gave on the Try for Dry Questionnaire, the records you kept in the Three-Day Diary, and any other information you may have obtained from your doctor, you will now select treatments from Table 5-1. Put a check mark next to the factors that you believe are contributing to your child's wetting. Then turn to the appropriate sections of this chapter for the information and instructions you will need to begin each treatment.

We recommend that all children who wet because of enuresis wear an enuresis alarm at night, in conjunction with the other treatments you have chosen from Table 5-1. *When used as part of a comprehensive treatment regime*, the enuresis alarm is the most effective tool available today. The alarm *by itself*, however, may not "cure" your child. As you now know, wetting is caused by a

TABLE 5-1. Quick Guide to Treatments

Cause	Treatment Section	Page
❑ Deep sleep	Arousing the Deep Sleeper	105
❑ Small bladder capacity; frequent urination	Increasing Bladder Capacity and Decreasing Urination Frequency	129
❑ Constipation; encopresis	Improving Bowel Health	147
❑ Food sensitivities	Tracking Problem Foods	155

number of factors. Deep sleep, for which the alarm is intended, is only one contributor. Keep in mind that your child is much more likely to reach dryness when several treatments are brought to bear simultaneously on the problem.

Reasons to Consider Delaying Treatment

Before you proceed to the descriptions of the Try for Dry treatments, we ask you to consider whether or not your family is ready for this plan. Prolonged periods of tension as a result of major changes in your family's life—or because of routine daily stresses—may interfere with your family's ability to follow through with a treatment program. Our program requires *consistency*. Stressed-out families may find it too difficult to comply with the program until things settle down in their lives.

As we have already mentioned, when the child has a psychological problem that could interfere with his progress, we usually recommend working with his doctor or psychologist to decide whether to postpone treatment for wetting. For example, children who are oppositional, psychotic, or antisocial should receive help for such problems before undertaking our plan.

TODDLERS NEED SPECIAL TREATMENT

Before starting an enuresis treatment for a toddler (that is, a child under five), remember that, by most definitions, night wetting before age five is normal and not diagnosed as enuresis. However, if you wish to help your younger child take some steps toward dryness, try simply building motivation and developing mental cues for dryness. Avoid using an enuresis alarm with a child younger than five: the noise may frighten a young child. Some common methods to try include the following:

- **Nightly routine.** Make sure that the child voids in the toilet before he goes to bed at night.
- **Positive practice.** Help the child get up from bed every night before he goes to sleep and practice going to the toilet.
- **Elimination diet.** Use the diet presented in Chapter 6 to isolate problem foods.
- **Positive reinforcement.** Give stickers or other valued rewards when the child stays dry.
- **Mental cues.** Talk with the child about staying dry, or have him draw pictures of himself getting up from bed to go to the bathroom at night.
- **Consultation with your doctor.** Ask your doctor about the possibility of using a medication for small bladder capacity.

Likewise, children with separation anxiety, who may fear sleeping away from home, may sabotage the program, intentionally or not, if their anxiety is not alleviated first. For example, one child we treated for enuresis just couldn't get to dry. Eventually we discovered that he was afraid of sleeping away from home. Because of his anxiety, he worried that if he became dry, he would no longer have an excuse to decline invitations to friends' homes. He dealt with this fear by disconnecting the alarm every night before he went to sleep, so that it would not sound when he wet. Once his fears came out, his parents reassured him: "Just because you're dry at night doesn't mean you *have* to sleep away from home." This reassurance permitted him to complete the program and get to dry.

Serious difficulties or major events in your family could hinder improvement as well. To determine whether or not there are any circumstances in your life that may call for postponing treatment, turn to the "Stressful Life Events Inventory" section of the questionnaire that you completed in Chapter 4 (see pages 77–78).

If you identified any events in the past year that have resulted in ongoing stress for your family, it is possible that, depending on the type of wetting your child is experiencing, this continued tension may (1) impair the resolution or treatment of her primary nocturnal enuresis, or (2) be the *cause* of her secondary enuresis, particularly if the wetting began shortly after a stressful event. The greater the number of stressful life events you have had, the greater the likelihood that they may have contributed to the wetting. Your child's enuresis may be evidence that she is having difficulty handling the events or their outcome. Carefully consider the effects that any of the following circumstances may be having on your child:

Death. If a significant person or family pet in your or your child's life has died, both you and your child may be struggling with grief. You may not have the needed motivation or enthusiasm to attack the wetting problem at this time. Keep in mind that the grieving process can take a year or even longer. So, until you and your child feel up to working on the tasks involved in our program, delay treatment.

Serious Illness. Taking care of a loved one who is ill may sap you of the necessary energy and attention you need to focus on treatment of your child's enuresis. Visits to the doctor, emergency trips to the hospital, and sleepless nights can result in your

GETTING IT ALL DOWN ON PAPER

If you suspect that everyday stresses may be affecting your child's wetting, try keeping a diary: Write down your child's description of the difficulties she encounters each day—at school, at home, and with her friends. Also write down any wetting episodes that occur on that day or night. After a week or so, look back in the diary. Were there any wet nights that followed very stressful days? If you find a pattern, consider talking to your child about her feelings. You may want to ask your pediatrician or school counselor for a referral to a psychotherapist (preferably someone experienced in treating enuresis). Once your child's life situation has improved, you may proceed with the treatment program.

emotional and physical exhaustion. Depending on the balance of your family's involvement with the ill person and your child's needs to get to dry, you will decide whether to wait or proceed with the plan.

Psychopathology. When, for instance, a sibling suffers from depression or ADHD, the disorder may distract parents from the job of consistently applying the techniques in our treatment program on the behalf of the enuretic child. When a parent has a psychological disorder, the parent may have difficulty being emotionally available, positive, and consistent in treating a child who wets. Even if one parent is psychologically healthy, he or she will likely be preoccupied with the spouse who is ill. So when a child's primary caretaker or other member of the family has a serious psychiatric problem (such as major depression, alcoholism or drug addiction, or psychosis) or displays abusive behavior, we recommend treatment for the troubled family member before trying to get the child to dry.

Birth of a Sibling. Secondary enuresis sometimes occurs with the arrival of a newborn in the home. A common conception is that a child who has begun to wet shortly after a new sibling is born does so in order to "get attention." This idea has not been examined scientifically. While we show here that there are many possible reasons why a child wets, when wetting follows a new birth, there are no clear explanations as to how this happens. No one understands whether the wetting is simply coincidental to the new birth or "caused" by it. So it is worth realizing that the public perception about this may or may not be accurate.

Exhausted parents of newborns certainly should not have to interrupt what little sleep they get to administer an enuresis treatment program for an older child. To stop the child's wetting, it may be enough to talk to your child about his feelings toward you and the new baby. Give him permission to be angry and to feel jealous of all the attention the baby is getting. Find opportunities to spend time alone with your older child and to reinforce "big kid" behavior. In time, your child may adjust to the new baby and return to dryness. If not, once the infant is sleeping through the night and the parents are well rested, your family will be in better condition to begin the program.

Financial or Work-Related Changes. When a parent loses a job, the entire family may feel significantly more stressed and worried. The loss of family income may force the other parent to start working outside the home while the unemployed parent faces the prospect of finding a new job, which may require different work hours, business travel, or even relocation. Parents often are tense during these periods of unemployment and may not have the patience or enthusiasm to focus on the wetting problem.

Not only losing a job, but also gaining a promotion can lead to increased tension at home. If a parent is promoted to a position that requires more work, more travel, or more responsibility, such a time may not be ideal for beginning treatment. On the other hand, a promotion or job change may increase income and reduce time away from home, thus reducing stress; such a development could be positive for the whole family and signal a good time to begin treatment.

If one parent has to work at night, the adult at home must be willing to undertake the responsibilities of the treatment program solo. If getting a full night's sleep is critical for the parent at home, it is preferable to wait until both parents' schedules allow them to be home at night. Single parents obviously do not have this option. If a single parent is to follow the program with a child, he or she must commit to several weeks or months (usually less than three) of consistent treatment, which will probably involve interrupted sleep.

School Changes. Let's say your family just moved to a new neighborhood, and now your child has started wetting at night. If talking about the move and working with school personnel to help the child integrate into the new school setting does not help the wetting remit over time, a family can begin treatment once everyone feels settled into their new home and community. If a child has primary enuresis, it is also better to wait until the child has adjusted to the new school setting before beginning the treatment program. If a child is having academic problems and needs a full night's sleep for optimal performance, it is probably better to wait until summer or a school winter or spring break to begin the treatment program.

Illicit Drug or Alcohol Use. A family member's substance abuse must be addressed and treated before you begin dryness treatment. Chemical dependency causes significant stress for all family members and may prevent parents from meeting the requirements of the program.

Parental Relationship. If you characterized your relationship with your spouse as mostly unhappy on the questionnaire in Chapter 4 (pages 76–79), it is possible that your marital difficulties are having a negative psychological effect on your child. This is particularly true if your child has secondary enuresis that began when the conflict or instability occurred at home. Your child may be aware of your unhappiness and concerned about either one or both of her parents. She may also be worried that her family might break up.

Your marital happiness may not be contributing to your child's wetting behavior, but it may weaken her ability to use the treatment consistently and so she may not get to dry. If the child sees you and your spouse fighting about her wetting, she may not have confidence in the treatment approach and may sabotage it with noncompliance. If your marital problems cause you and your spouse to make power plays out of parenting decisions, we recommend couples therapy. An improved domestic relationship can only help your child. *You and your spouse must resolve any disagreements about this program before treatment begins.*

IF YOUR FAMILY is in the midst of any stressful situations, discuss them with your child and find out how he feels. If talking about the issues and trying to resolve them does not decrease or stop the wetting, seek professional counseling before proceeding, particularly if your child has secondary enuresis.

After you have considered the results of your inventory of stressful life events and after you have determined that this is a good time to pursue enuresis treatments, acquaint yourself with the use of the enuresis alarm. Then, you should read about the appropriate treatments that target the causes of wetting that you identified in Chapter 4.

Arousing the Deep Sleeper: The Enuresis Alarm

BASIC PRINCIPLES

The enuresis alarm is a device that sets off a bell, buzzer, or other noisemaker when a child begins to wet. Originally wired together from a modified mattress pad and an electric doorbell, the enuresis alarm has been in use since about 1940. Today's modern alarms hardly resemble the original. As shown in Figure 5-1 (see page 114), enuresis alarms sold nowadays are easy to operate and smaller than a pager. They consist of a moisture sensor—a pair of metal strips or a metal snap—that attaches to the child's underpants and a sounding mechanism, such as a buzzer or vibrator.

The enuresis device, which on average costs about eighty dollars, works mechanically in the following way: Because urine contains electrolytes, urine conducts electricity; so, if urine touches the metal strips of the alarm sensor, it completes a microcircuit in the device, allowing the tiny electrical current created with the battery to sound the alarm.

As we have said, there are many types of enuresis alarms on the market. At minimum, a good alarm will respond quickly to moisture and sound loudly enough to wake a parent sleeping nearby. We prefer alarms with sounding devices that are worn on the pajama shoulder so the alarm is close to the child's ear. The sound from devices worn on the waist can be hard to hear because it tends to be muffled by blankets. Alarms that just vibrate in response to wetting do not awaken the parent.

The sensors in contemporary alarms are quite sensitive; when the child begins to wet they require very little moisture to make the buzzer sound. The bell, which can be as small as an earring box, is powered by a button-size battery similar to those used in hearing aids. Some alarms are affixed to the child's underwear with Velcro straps or worn on the wrist like a watch.

Although the bell and mattress pad device is still available, it is certainly no longer the best choice for treatment. With this older type of alarm, the child must wet through his bedclothes onto and through the sheets before the moisture reaches the wire mesh mattress pad and causes the alarm to go off. If the child rolls off the pad entirely or wets while sleeping on his back, the pad may not get wet at all when the voiding occurs. Also, this type of alarm is more likely than the newer alarms to sound in response to perspiration.

HOW DOES THE ENURESIS ALARM WORK?

Good question. We thought you'd like to know. So would we. Actually, there is no consensus among health professionals on the precise mechanism at work when an alarm helps a child stop wetting. So, rather than compare several theories and risk sounding like a textbook, we will present the explanation that we think is most likely the correct one.

The enuresis alarm seems to stop bedwetting through "training." Teaching or training an alert person to change his behavior is easy enough. In the case of bedwetting, the challenge is to control the wetting behavior that occurs while a child is asleep. The alarm is necessary because the child sleeps so deeply that she cannot perceive an impending bladder contraction or the sense of urgency it creates. Her bladder contracts without her awareness or attempt to stop it. Treatment with an alarm attempts to break that chain of events by "training" the child to sense an impending contraction and get up to urinate.

We use the following explanation to understand how the

alarm usually helps to bring about a change in behavior from wetting to dryness. (The explanation also works when the alarm is used in the daytime to control day wetting.)

1. During the night, as the child's bladder fills with urine, it tends to contract.

2. Because the child sleeps so deeply, he does not sense the contraction and so cannot inhibit it. He begins to wet.

3. The first drops of urine cause the alarm to sound as a "bladder burglar alarm," but the deeply asleep child does not respond to the noise or to the wetness. [The drug Ditropan (see "Oxybutynin, page 130) is a component of the Try for Dry program that is very helpful in keeping this first release of urine to just a spot; much urine still remains in the bladder.]

4. A family member—a "deputy bladder police officer," if you will—responds to the "burglar alarm" by taking the child to the toilet, trying to awaken him (but not necessarily succeeding). If you are able to awaken your child, you may find that learning dryness will be achieved faster. But if you can't rouse him, don't be frustrated; it's often next to impossible to wake a deep sleeper. Be satisfied in the meantime to get him to the toilet before his bladder is completely empty.

   Although there are various ideas about what a parent should do when the alarm sounds, one thing you should not do is simply stay in bed. You should rush to the child's room and take him to the toilet, whether you manage to awaken him or not. Do use gentle measures, such as turning on the lights in the room or saying "Please, get up—the alarm's gone off," in trying to awaken your child. Avoid harsh measures, such as slapping or screaming.

5. The child finishes urinating in the toilet and then goes back to bed.

6. Eventually, the repetition of this procedure conditions the child to associate the urge to urinate with the need to go to the toilet. After a few weeks of going to the bathroom every time the alarm sounds, the child will begin to "tune in" to his bladder while asleep. He also will begin to develop the skill of inhibiting the release of urine.

Perhaps an analogy with stroke patients is helpful toward understanding how such training may awaken dormant portions of our nervous system. When an adult experiences a stroke, which results in a portion of the brain becoming incapacitated due to a lack of blood flow, the segment of the body served by this portion of the brain loses its function. Perhaps an arm may be paralyzed or a leg may fail to support walking. The brain cannot regrow or reconstruct this lost segment. So, how can physical and occupational therapists bring about such good results in stroke victims, simply by having their patients repeatedly do specific exercises that focus on "retraining" the affected arm or leg?

In the case of stroke victims, we believe that the central nervous system has "back-up" nerve bundles that are "dormant" and come to be "enlisted" and "aroused" by the process of physical therapy. In a similar manner, the enuresis alarm may encourage the brain to arouse dormant or immature nerve bundles, which now permit the children to inhibit a nighttime bladder contraction or arouse themselves to use the toilet. Perhaps, in the case of children who "outgrow" the bedwetting without any treatment, this "arousal" occurs naturally and is what happens when we think of them as "matured."

Once the training process is under way, about half of the children who use the alarm get out of bed themselves and walk to the toilet to urinate. The other half seem to start inhibiting their bladder contraction, so they do not get up at all at night.

In time, the children who have been walking to the toilet at night learn to inhibit the release of urine for longer and longer durations. Ultimately, most children who follow the alarm routine end up staying in bed all night rather than getting up to urinate. After about eight weeks of alarm use, the typical child should have an improved record of dryness at night; by about twelve weeks, most children should have complete bladder control all night long.

Will the enuresis alarm end bedwetting for every child? No, but it will for the majority of children, when it is used *consistently and in conjunction with the other treatments* in this book. It will *not* correct wetting in cases of incontinence or of primary sleep disorder, or in the relatively rare instances in which deep sleep is not a factor in the child's wetting.

WHY HASN'T THE ALARM BEEN MORE POPULAR IN THE PAST?

In the existing medical research, the enuresis alarm has consistently achieved the best success record in helping children get to dry. But paradoxically, using an alarm is the least popular approach. Here are some reasons why it is not used more widely, followed by explanations to counter such concerns.

The Most Common Reasons People Reject the Alarm

1. *It takes too long.* In our "quick fix" society, many people are impatient with a treatment that takes significant time and effort—especially in the middle of the night! It may be easier to have your child "take a pill" or to just ignore the wetting, hoping that it will go away.

   Counter. While it is true that when used *alone*, the alarm method may take six months to work, when the alarm is used consistently in conjunction with our Try for Dry program, children show improved dryness much more quickly, commonly within a few weeks.

2. *Alarms are unfamiliar to many health-care professionals and most parents.* Even more than fifty years after the first alarm's introduction, the medical community at large still has little personal experience with the enuresis alarm, so doctors may not readily suggest using it.

Counter. We anticipate that wider appreciation of successful alarm use will make it more familiar.

3. *Parents may be apprehensive that, by focusing attention on their child's genitalia every night at bedtime, they are sending him some kind of negative unconscious message.* Because of this concern, they may just instinctively reject the idea of attaching a mechanical device near their child's genital area.

Counter. While parents are entitled to their apprehensions, there is no evidence that affixing such a device to the underpants causes psychological harm.

4. *Parents may fear that their child could choke himself on the wire.*

Counter. To our knowledge, no child has ever choked or injured himself with the enuresis alarm.

5. *To some, the theory behind the enuresis alarm is illogical because it is believed that learning is supposed to happen by avoiding the undesirable behavior or activity.* If the alarm sounds after the wetting happens—after it's "too late"—how can a child learn not to wet at night?

Counter. Logic aside, alarm usage seems to work. Here's why we think it does. Because alarm sounding is *not* paired with voiding (that is, the complete emptying of the bladder), rather, because it is paired with the *brief* release of only a *small* volume of urine, the child does eventually learn dryness. The alarm sounds while there is still time either for her to be taken to the toilet to void or to inhibit a bladder contraction. Additionally, we believe that parental praise and reinforcement during the training assists in this learning process.

6. *People may hear stories from neighbors or friends about unsuccessful treatments using the alarm.* "It woke everybody in the house except William. He just slept right through it."

Counter. These stories abound when families have not been taught the correct use of the alarm. Their child likely will sleep through the noise, but after repeated awakenings by the parents, dryness will be attained.

Although each of these concerns is legitimate, the effectiveness of the enuresis alarm is overwhelming. No single treatment, *when used properly,* has as good a success rate in curing wetting as the enuresis alarm, particularly in the case of bedwetting. The likelihood of getting dry is even stronger when alarm use is coordinated with the use of reinforcements (see "Reinforcement," pages 162–168). Additionally, when the alarm is used consistently in conjunction with other treatments, the success occurs faster.

TREATMENT INSTRUCTIONS

1. **Obtain an alarm.** Once you have obtained an enuresis alarm, follow the instructions included with the device. (For information on where you can purchase an alarm, see Appendix D.) *Note:* Your insurance carrier may reimburse you for all or part of the cost of the device, as it is common to reimburse subscribers for the purchase of "durable" medical equipment. A prescription is not currently needed to obtain an alarm, but

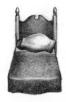

INTRODUCING THE ALARM TO YOUR CHILD

Because the sound of the enuresis alarm may frighten a young child, we typically do not advise the use of an alarm for children under five years old. If you do want to try the alarm treatment with your young child, however, be sure to spend some extra time familiarizing her with the alarm.

Before using the alarm at night, first gradually introduce loud sounds. For example, have the child shout loudly, then play a music selection loudly, then ask if it is OK for you to shout loudly. Then both of you should shout loudly. *Then* sound the alarm. By comparison, the loud alarm noise may then sound less frightening to the child.

Also, try playing a game of making other loud sounds together, like turning the radio volume up and talking loudly to one another before sounding the alarm, so that the first few times the child hears the alarm its relative volume is not as great as when it suddenly goes off in a quiet room. Once the child has heard the alarm a few times, she will know what to expect and should not be afraid of it.

Then let her touch the moisture sensor with wet fingertips so that she can control when the sound of the alarm will occur. If the child continues to be afraid of the alarm, let her put it on her favorite stuffed animal or doll. Or, ask an older sibling to model it. Then make the alarm sound—by moistening the sensor—as if the alarm wearer had wet. Ask the fearful child to help the sibling (or stuffed animal or doll) "who just wet" not to be scared. Give messages of encouragement and coping, such as "Don't be afraid" and "It's just a loud noise."

If these techniques fail to help your child accept an enuresis alarm, you may choose to adopt other treatment approaches. (See "Scheduled Lifting: An Alternative Approach," page 116.)

your insurance transactions may be expedited if your doctor provides you with a signed prescription for the device.

2. **Test the alarm.** To test an alarm, pinch the moisture sensor between your fingertips. The alarm should sound. If it doesn't,

check the batteries. Also, some devices have a plastic tab inserted by the manufacturer in order to prevent discharge of the batteries. In order for the device to sound, you must pull the plastic tab out.

3. **Attach the alarm.** As shown in Figure 5-1, you should attach the alarm's moisture sensor to your child's underpants. Carefully place the sensor where the child's urine is likely to dampen it: For girls, attach it low on the front panel of the underpants; for boys, it should go slightly higher.

In using the alarm, watch for any shearing of the wire at its junction with the alarm box. If your child is rough, consider putting a piece of electrical tape over this spot to reinforce the connection.

THE ALARM SCHEDULE

It is very important for your child to wear the enuresis alarm *consistently*. In order for the alarm to be effective, your child should comply with the following schedule:

Step 1. The child should wear the alarm *every night* until he has fourteen consecutive dry days and nights.

Step 2. After fourteen days and nights of dryness, the child may wear the alarm *every other night* for two weeks.

- If the child wets no more than once during this two-week period, go on to step 3.
- If the child has more than one wet night in the two-week period, immediately return to step 1 and repeat the process.

Step 3. The child may now wear the alarm every third night for two weeks.

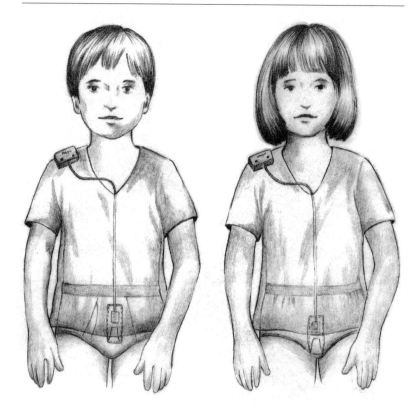

Figure 5-1. For nighttime use the enuresis alarm is attached low on the front panel of the child's underpants. It is positioned slightly higher for boys than it is for girls.

- If the child wets no more than once during this two-week period, go on to step 4.
- If the child has more than one wet night in the two-week period, immediately return to step 1 and repeat the process.

Step 4. The child may now wear the alarm every fourth night for two weeks.

- If the child has no more than one wet night in the two-week period, go on to step 5.

- If the child has more than one wet night in the two-week period, immediately return to step 1 and repeat the process.

Step 5. Discontinue using the alarm. Taper off from the other concurrent treatments, as described in Chapter 8 (pages 177–180).

Many families we see in our practice are so frustrated with their child's wetting problem that just starting the alarm treatment for them is like seeing the light at the end of a dark tunnel. We tell them to expect their child to begin having dry nights after using the enuresis alarm for one month. If their child responds to the alarm and the accompanying treatments (given in Chapter 6) in one month's time, then continuing the treatments should lead to dryness. If, on the other hand, their child shows no progress in one month, they should talk to their doctor and fine-tune the program. (It is also possible that your child has not yet shown dryness because he is experiencing incontinence, not enuresis.) To help parents get past any reluctance they may have about the amount of work involved in this treatment, we stress that this first month is a "trial period." Taking the program one step at a time will improve everyone's outlook, reduce the level of stress associated with wetting, and increase your child's chances for success.

PRACTICAL ADVICE

In this section, we offer some tips involving alarm use that you should consider in the light of day, as you prepare for the sounding of the alarm at night:

You and your spouse need to agree in advance which one of you will get up with the child each night. Ideally, the enuresis alarm would

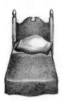

SCHEDULED LIFTING:
AN ALTERNATIVE APPROACH

Experts agree: Deep sleep, or better, the failure to arouse from sleep, is the major factor in bedwetting. If your child sleeps so heavily that a shrieking smoke detector won't wake him, then neither will a full bladder.

However, if you and your family decide, for whatever reason, that the enuresis alarm is not for you, one alternative is literally to lift the child out of bed and carry him to the toilet every night. This is also called encouraged voiding. In theory, such repetitive activity will eventually become a habit for the child. The child will "learn" in his sleep, as it were. He will come to arouse himself from sleep to go to the toilet, or else he will unconsciously inhibit a naturally impending bladder contraction during sleep.

Knowing when to lift depends on when the wetting happens. For many children, wetting occurs about one-half to one hour after bedtime, then again at about 11:00 P.M., 2:00 A.M., and 5:00 A.M. In other words, it may occur about four times per night. (When a child spontaneously outgrows enuresis, the wetting seems to stop first at the period shortly after sleep. Then there appears to be a reduction in the volume of wetting at 11:00 P.M. and 2:00 A.M. Next, the wetting ceases at 11:00 P.M., then at 2:00 A.M., then finally at 5:00 A.M.) Using this pattern as a guide, you might check your child throughout the night for a few nights to determine when wetting is happening.

If you are able to ascertain a pattern in your child's wetting, then

rouse the sleeping child: he would get up and urinate in the toilet and then return to bed, all without assistance. In reality, very often a child who wets sleeps too deeply to respond to the alarm. So, it falls to the parents or other adult family members to listen for the alarm as a "sentry" during their sleep and, when it does go off, to get up and help the child to the toilet. If possible, arrange to alternate turns with your spouse, so that each of you can at least get a good night's sleep every other night.

try a preemptive lifting. Carry your child to the toilet about fifteen minutes before you expect wetting to happen. Lift him to the toilet even if he is not fully awake. Doing this every night may be enough to reduce the amount and frequency of the wetting. Over the next few weeks, you'll find out if you're making progress. This strategy seems to work in about 10 percent of children who bedwet.

If you find that your child wets a short time after you've lifted him, try not to be frustrated with yourself or your child. Some families fear that there must be a medical problem—such as a blockage of the bladder—because their child wets soon after an encouraged void. They may think, "If he just urinated in the toilet and didn't drink anything and then wets his bed, he can't be emptying his bladder when I lift him." Actually, this pattern of wetting shortly after an encouraged void is common. It likely relates to the cyclical nature of bladder contractions, which the child has not yet learned to inhibit. It may also relate to how the body handles a water-retaining hormone, vasopressin [see "Overproduction of Urine at Night (Polyuria)," page 144].

Lifting may work for milder cases of bedwetting, but it is not practical for parents who are unable to stand vigil through the night. Also, it can be physically difficult to do if the child is older, or heavier, or both. Finally, a theoretical problem with this tactic is that since you cannot accurately predict the time at which the child's bladder will be full, this method may not teach the child to wake himself when he needs to urinate. So, while scheduled lifting is cheap and worth a try, don't be disappointed if it doesn't work.

Avoid asking an older sibling to assume responsibility for getting up with the child at night. Whenever possible, arrange to be home when your child is wearing the alarm at night. It is a parent's responsibility to manage the child's treatment. A sibling who is made to stand in for a parent could come to resent his or her brother or sister for wetting, as well as the parents for not taking charge. Also, by following through on your commitment to help your child stop wetting, you send a powerful message to all of your children.

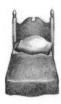

STAYING WITH IT

Making sure that your child uses the enuresis alarm every night—and follows the other treatments you have chosen as well—can be challenging. From our experience, we have learned that the number one enemy of progress toward dryness is not being compliant with the program.

Most kids seem to hate routines that are imposed on them, especially if they don't understand the reason behind a new regimen. So, make sure your child sees the connection between faithful use of the alarm and permanent dryness. Explain that, just like learning to play a musical instrument, she has to practice every day—even when she doesn't feel like it. If she wants to get dry, she needs to follow the schedule.

If your child has too many wetting episodes while tapering alarm use and has to return to step 1 in the alarm schedule, try to reassure her. Explain that starting over is not a punishment, but simply what needs to be done to make sure that the alarm is teaching her bladder control well. Beginning again at step 1, after weeks of progress, can be the most difficult part of the process—for both children and parents. This is the time when a well-chosen reward or other motivational device can really do wonders in helping to prop up a child's sagging commitment (see Chapter 7).

Ultimately, your participation and faith in the program may be your child's primary motivation for staying with it. If your child balks at the program at first, you must resist the natural temptation to give up. Encouraging your child to continue is the most important part you can play in the successful resolution of this problem.

The child should sleep in a room near your bedroom, if possible, to make it easier for you to hear and respond to the alarm. Because you will probably be getting up with your child, it is a good idea to have your rooms close together. As we have seen, most children with enuresis are deep sleepers. The sound of the enuresis alarm will most likely wake you before it wakes your child, at least in the beginning. When the alarm goes off, you need to be close enough to hear it and get to your child quickly to lead him to the toilet before his bladder is completely empty. Note, though, that the child should not sleep in the *same* room as you: doing so could reinforce the wetting problem, since most children enjoy having a parent stay with them. Additionally, children can become dependent on sleeping near a parent, which may end up harming a child's self-concept, particularly if the child sees himself as being immature.

If it is impossible or impractical to be nearby, consider using a baby monitor or an intercom, which will enable you to hear what is going on in your child's room. With this arrangement, when the alarm sounds you will be able to hear it easily. If a sibling must move out of his or her bedroom so that the child who wets can be closer to you, explain to the displaced brother or sister that this is a temporary arrangement and that he or she will move back when the enuretic child is dry.

If possible, have your child sleep in the bedroom closest to the bathroom. The shorter the distance your child has to travel at night, the better the chance that she will make it in time to complete her urination. It is also safer if she does not have to walk very far in a sleepy condition.

Make sure the route to the bathroom is clear of toys and other obstacles and is also adequately lit with nightlights. There are a variety of inexpensive nightlights that plug into electrical sockets and are bright enough to illuminate a path without keeping anyone awake. Some models turn themselves on when the natural lighting is dim and turn themselves off when the room brightens, so that you can keep them plugged in all day. Putting a nightlight in the bathroom is nice, too, so that the child does not have to face harsh, bright lights when she gets up to urinate.

Make sure your child's room, or at least his bed, stays comfortably warm through the night. It's a common, though unexplained, phenomenon: As soon as you step out into the cold after being in a warm room, you get the urge to relieve your bladder. For children who are particularly sensitive to cold, wetting is sometimes worse in winter months because of the same phenomenon. One family reported that after they installed a heater in their child's previously cold waterbed, the wetting stopped. For another child, simply moving the bed away from a cold, exposed bedroom wall reduced the wetting.

Organize your child's room to make nighttime cleanup more convenient. Since your child will continue to wet while learning to improve her bladder control, it is a good idea to keep fresh bed sheets, pajamas, and underwear in the child's room. In fact, because many children wet more than once a night, having two or more sets of bedding and clothing at hand is advisable. Also, as long as your child is comfortable with the idea, consider putting a hamper or basket in the child's room to receive the soiled laundry. If the child wants to keep her wetting private, she can remove the hamper from her room when she is expecting visitors.

Be sure that your child follows a similar alarm procedure wherever he sleeps. In families with multiple households, because of divorce or other reasons, the child must either take his alarm with him or have an additional alarm at his other home. Continuity is key to his becoming dry. Similarly, if your child routinely sleeps at his grandparents' house, make sure that everyone understands the alarm procedure. (You may want to share this book with the adult who will be responsible for your child when he is away.)

Using the Enuresis Alarm During the Day

If your child has diurnal enuresis, that is, if your child wets during the day, he can still benefit from the alarm program. If he has greater than normal urination frequency or urgency, first make sure that she is evaluated by a physician or pediatric urologist. If your child is diagnosed with enuresis, not incontinence, you may start a daytime alarm regimen. Before you begin, however, sit down with your child and make a list of priorities with him. Which is more important, bladder control or soccer? Bladder control or Little League? If your child participates in many after-school activities, consider curtailing some of them for a while. If bladder control is high enough on your child's list, and you are willing to commit your time and effort to the program, proceed with the following steps:

Step 1. For two weeks, have your child put on the alarm at home, every day, at a regular, agreed-upon time: say, when she comes home from school and on weekends. She should wear the alarm initially for at least four hours a day in the first week. If your child's bladder capacity is low, your doctor may prescribe a bladder medication, Ditropan, to reduce the wetting. Your child should make regular trips to the toilet while wearing the alarm. You should use a chart to monitor voiding and dryness and to use stickers and other reinforcers to reward progress (see "Rewarding Daytime Dryness," page 167).

- If your child wets infrequently, perhaps one to two times a day, you can reward her with a sticker for staying dry for extended intervals, such as a half day or the whole day.
- If she wets frequently—more than two times per day—have her visit the toilet to try to void every two

hours, and reward her if she is able to "Beat the Buzzer" and stay dry during that interval. As dryness becomes more consistent, extend the intervals by an hour at a time.

Step 2. In the second week, increase the amount of time your child wears the alarm before and up to bedtime (for example, from 4:00 to 9:00 P.M.).

Step 3. See how it goes. The more time your child wears the alarm, the more learning opportunities he will have. Note that this daytime training is so effective because it offers so many training opportunities. A child who drinks a moderate amount of liquid and wears the alarm throughout the day will have many chances to improve.

PRACTICAL ADVICE

Some children respond well to making a game of it. In addition to playing "Beat the Buzzer," your child can have fun learning to control his bladder by wearing the alarm on his belt and referring to it as a "bladder pager." The medication oxybutynin can make the learning easier, because it reduces the sense of urgency and "slows" bladder contractions (see "Oxybutynin," page 130).

Working on day wetting and night wetting problems simultaneously may be too much of a strain on your family. Most prefer to treat the day wetting first, because it interferes more with the child's social activities. Other families see "dry" results quickly and are happy to treat both day and night wetting simultaneously.

The child should never wear the "noise" alarm to school, because it would cause her embarrassment. However, please use your judgment about using the noise alarm in other public places. If you feel that the alarm sounding would not embarrass your child in your backyard, for example, or riding in your car with the family,

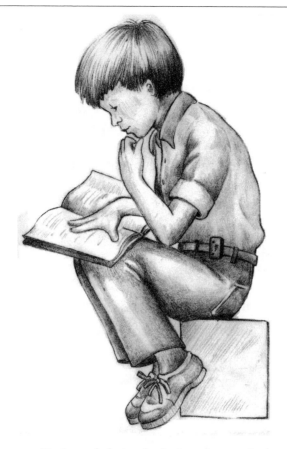

Figure 5-2. For intervals during the daytime, the enuresis alarm can be worn on a child's belt like a "pager."

then consider these times opportunities to further the training process. Otherwise, if you want to extend the learning sessions outside the home but keep the sessions private, you could use an alarm that vibrates (see Appendix D). Another helpful way to keep up the training is to arrange a timed voiding schedule for her to follow while she is at school (see "A Voiding Schedule," page 141).

Be very careful about how you respond to your child's "accidents."
If you make a big production out of changing the wet child or
yell at your child, you may actually reinforce the behavior. That
is, because the child gets special or extra attention when he wets
(even though it may be negative attention), he may continue to
wet. Instead, when your child wets, respond neutrally, in a mat-
ter-of-fact manner. By all means, support and encourage your
child to be responsible for changing his clothes and rinsing them
out in the sink, when appropriate. But try not to draw too much
attention to the wetting.

Summary

In this chapter we have presented the method for choosing your
child's treatment plan, and we have described the most important tool at your disposal for ending wetting: the enuresis alarm.
In the next chapter, you will learn about the other components
of the Try for Dry plan, some or all of which you will use, in
conjunction with the alarm, to help your child reach his or her
goal of dryness.

Questions and Answers

Q: *We have four children—ages four to twelve—and three bed-
rooms in our house. The oldest wets his bed about once a week. But
he shares a bunk bed with his younger brother, so I'm reluctant to
try the alarm because it'll probably wake everyone up. Do you have
any suggestions?*

A: If the child who wets wants to work on his wetting but waking up the entire household is a problem, try moving the child

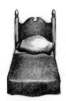

DON'T TRY THESE AT HOME

According to the article "An Historical Account of Enuresis," by Lucille Glicklich, humans have been trying to cure enuresis since at least 1550 B.C. The ancient Greeks concocted their remedies from such ingredients as juniper berries, cyprus, and beer. In the West African kingdom of Dahomey, the initial treatment for children who wet was a beating. If enuresis persisted, the child was humiliated by being doused with a mixture of water and ashes and driven into the street, where other children would jeer, "Adida ga ga ga ga," which means "Urine everywhere."

Over the years, children have endured harsh ritualistic treatments, such as spikes and ropes in their beds, as well as elevation of the feet and pelvis while sleeping. In the nineteenth and early twentieth centuries, catheterization and a variety of external devices were also presumed to stop enuresis.

None of these remedies is recommended today.

to another room temporarily. If that is not a realistic option, here are a few others:

- Scheduled lifting
- Mild fluid restriction
- Positive practice in toileting before bed
- Monitoring bladder capacity by diary to see if it is reduced
- The medication Ditropan

Another alternative is to try the medication called DDAVP. (We talk more about this and other medications and options in Chapter 6.)

Q: *How dependable is the enuresis alarm? Can I count on it to work every time?*

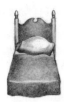

THE TRY FOR DRY SONG

In our practice, we've created a song especially for children with verses that express optimism about reaching dryness. Since we've found that the song is fun and motivating for young children, we will include the appropriate verses from the song in each major treatment section of the book. The music and lyrics to the song in its entirety appear in Appendix B.

VERSE 1

Bladder high, / bladder low, / bladder full, / I gotta go.

Refrain
I'm gonna try, / Try for Dry, / and when I do, / I'm gonna be / mighty high!

VERSE 2

I'm gonna try, AT NIGHT, / to feel my pee. / But, Mister Sleep's / distractin' me.

I've gotta work / to get him off o' me. / OFF O' ME! / So's I can be / dry for me!

Refrain
I'm gonna try, / Try for Dry, / and when I do, / I'm gonna be / mighty high!

A: Naturally, the alarm will go off every time the sensors are moistened, but is it guaranteed to "work" to correct bedwetting in every child? No. The alarm will not stop wetting when a child has incontinence, when a child has a primary sleep disorder, or when it is used inconsistently, and it only occasionally works when deep sleep is not a contributor to wetting. For the *majority* of bedwetting cases, however, deep sleep and small bladder capacity are the causative factors. Coexisting problems of bowel irregularity and food sensitivities are less frequently noted. So, the enuresis alarm, in concert with other appropriate treatments described in Chapter 6, will resolve wetting when used correctly.

Q: *Should I put my child in underpants or Pull-Ups at night?*

A: The best answer to this question depends on the reaction of the child to the wetting. If the child doesn't really want to get up from bed to void, then it sounds as if you aren't going to make progress treating the bedwetting anyway, so it doesn't matter. Pull-Ups are easier and give you and your washing machine a break from extra laundry. On the other hand, if you are going to be using an enuresis alarm anyway, you may choose to permit the child to wear the alarm—affixed to the underwear—and put the Pull-Up *over* the underwear. Be careful, though, because Pull-Ups can be so effective at wicking urine away from the sensor that the sensor may not moisten, and the alarm will not sound even if the child wets.

In addition, having the child wear both Pull-Ups and the alarm may be sending mixed messages that could decrease the motivation to get to dry. If your child is not making progress while wearing Pull-Ups, we recommend refraining from using them.

Chapter 6

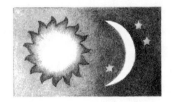

Helper Treatments

IN THE PREVIOUS chapter, we asked you to choose the treatments for your child's wetting based on the contributing factors you and your doctor have observed. Then we presented the first and most important regimen for getting to dry: arousing the deep sleeper with the enuresis alarm. In this chapter, we give detailed instructions for counteracting the three remaining major factors that are likely to hinder getting dry: (1) small functional bladder capacity, (2) constipation and bowel irregularity, and (3) food sensitivities. Refer to Table 6-1 to find each treatment. (If your child is younger than five years old, make sure you have read "Toddlers Need Special Treatment," page 99, before continuing. As we point out there, we usually recommend delaying the use of the enuresis alarm or medication in children younger than five.)

TABLE 6-1. Quick Guide to Treatments

Cause	Treatment Section	Page
❑ Small bladder capacity; frequent urination	Increasing Bladder Capacity and Decreasing Urination Frequency	129
❑ Constipation; encopresis	Improving Bowel Health	147
❑ Food sensitivities	Tracking Problem Foods	155

Increasing Bladder Capacity and Decreasing Urination Frequency

SMALL BLADDER CAPACITY

"From the Three-Day Diary you completed, Mrs. Jones, your eight-year-old boy shows a bladder capacity of five ounces. In other words, your boy has the same bladder capacity as a three-year-old."

Most children who bedwet have a functional bladder capacity that is smaller than normal; only a minority of children who bedwet have a normal or greater than normal bladder capacity. So, small functional bladder capacity is likely to slow your child's progress toward dryness. Because this treatment for small bladder capacity involves taking a medication dispensed by prescription, you will need to consult your doctor before proceeding. This is especially important if your child also has a history of urine infection or day wetting. Show the doctor your Three-Day Diary, and discuss your conclusions about your child's bladder capacity. If you need to add this treatment to your child's program, follow the instructions below, and keep your doctor informed of your child's progress.

Oxybutynin

Oxybutynin (trade name Ditropan) is a medication commonly prescribed to treat day wetness. By itself, with no other simultaneous treatment, oxybutynin has not proven effective in treating bedwetting. But when this medication plays a supporting role, as a "helper" to the main treatment (the alarm), oxybutynin is very beneficial. The families in our Try for Dry program have often reported that the medication seemed to help their children get dry permanently. Some families tell us:

"Gee, I think the medicine got him dry . . . He used to use the bathroom so often in the daytime, and we measured how small his bladder was."

Other families tell us:

"Gee, I think the alarm did it; he was just so sleepy."

Either way, the medication seems to be beneficial, and the children get to dry.

Why might oxybutynin work? There are three likely reasons: (1) it reduces the sense of urgency that children feel when the bladder is about to contract, (2) it reduces the intensity, or strength, of bladder contractions, and (3) it prolongs the time it takes the bladder to empty. Before taking oxybutynin, a child may have a "brittle" bladder—in other words, it may empty when it holds only a small volume of urine, and do it so quickly that the child does not have the time even to sense the contraction. Once the medication is used, however, a child who wets by day will likely now be able to sense the bladder contraction before it's too late—or at least have enough time to try delaying the contraction either by inhibiting the bladder muscle or tightening his external sphincter. In the case of night wetting, oxybu-

NAME _____   AGE_____

ADDRESS _____

_____   DATE _____

$\mathcal{R}_\chi$ **TRY FOR DRY**

DITROPAN: SYRUP (5mg/5ml)
            or TABLETS (5mg)

        Sig:

        Disp:

CAUTION: May cause problematic dry mouth, blurred
vision, constipation, upset stomach, or nasal irritation.
A flushed face may appear and should not be a problem.

❏ LABEL

REFILL   1   2   3   4   PRN   NR

DEA# _____   _____M.D.

tynin (when used with the alarm program) seems to give parents
a bit more time to respond to the alarm. So when they bring the
child to the toilet, the bladder is not totally empty, and the child
can void on the toilet. And the bed may only get damp instead

of soaked. So oxybutynin gives everyone some much needed breathing room while the child "learns" to master his bladder.

For children with small bladder capacity who are dry by day but wet at night, taking small doses of oxybutynin during the day as well as at bedtime has proved helpful in alleviating the nighttime wetting. (For the 10 percent of children who wet only at night but have normal bladder capacity, oxybutynin may not be helpful.) Your doctor needs to evaluate your child's bladder capacity before prescribing the medication for this purpose.

Families may be reluctant to choose medication treatments for their children because they are apprehensive about short- or long-term side effects of the medication. If you have such concerns, discuss them with your doctor. One common additional effect of oxybutynin is red cheeks, which is caused by the relaxation of the smooth muscles that cover the blood vessels in the face. This effect is usually harmless, although in the summer months, children may feel slightly overheated because of it. In fact, this effect is so predictable that doctors sometimes judge the effectiveness of oxybutynin by looking for red cheeks. If the child has shown no improvement after a month of taking oxybutynin and her cheeks are not red, perhaps a higher dose is warranted. In any case, it is rare for a family to be so apprehensive about oxybutynin that they decide against it. In our experience, it is an effective, safe medication.

Oxybutynin may actually increase bladder capacity over many months' time. Remember, though, that becoming dry at night depends not so much on how big the bladder is, but rather on how well the child can sense and inhibit an imminent bladder contraction during sleep. Children with normal bladder capacity who usually do not wet may do so under special circumstances (if they are overtired, if they overdrink, and so on). So, children who become dry while taking only oxybutynin without other

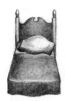

NOT RECOMMENDED: IMIPRAMINE

A medication that has been widely used to treat children with bedwetting is an antidepressant called imipramine—sold most commonly under the trade name of Tofranil. This medication appears to cause the depth of sleep to be "shallower," and so may permit children to inhibit their impending bladder contraction. The drug also has some effects on the bladder itself similar to oxybutynin, and may promote enlargement of bladder capacity.

Imipramine has a very serious downside, however: overdoses can be fatal. The drug must be kept in a locked cabinet out of children's reach at all times.

Other adverse effects reported by families include sleeplessness and resulting fatigue, weight loss, and temporary hair loss. Like all of the drug therapies we are aware of, imipramine used alone may have some short-term benefits, but most children wet again when they stop taking it.

Our advice is to stay clear of imipramine as a treatment for enuresis because the negative factors outweigh possible benefits. If your physician prescribes imipramine for your child's enuresis, be sure to ask why he chose this drug and not another. If you are not satisfied, get another opinion.

treatments may wet again once they stop taking the medication. In the majority of cases, when prescribed properly, oxybutynin will enable the child with a small functional bladder capacity to hold urine more effectively, thereby improving her chances to be successful with other treatments.

Children with typical bedwetting who take oxybutynin in conjunction with the alarm, the bowel program, and the Happy Bladder Diet, as described in this book, come to show new dryness within a month and usually remission of wetting by three months. When one component of that plan is omitted—say, the medication—dryness will come a lot more slowly, possibly in six

NOT RECOMMENDED: SEVERE RESTRICTION OF LIQUIDS IN THE EVENING

It seems like a natural solution: If we drink less, we expect to urinate less. So why not withhold all liquids after dinner from a child who wets?

Well, there is a minimum amount of urine the body needs to excrete, regardless of the amount we drink. Drinking less does result in less urine being excreted, but the bladder may still fill with enough urine to cause the bladder to contract. Also, a child's pituitary gland may not be making enough of the urine-concentrating hormone vasopressin. So despite very little intake of fluids, the child may still make too much urine at night.

months. Because it can take so long to see results this way, many families conclude that the plan doesn't work and give up trying after a month of treatment. Keep this in mind when you are considering whether or not to choose oxybutynin (see the section below). Also remember that your child's initial successes will greatly influence his and your outlook. Without medication, progress toward dryness may be so slow that "failure" is likely. On the other hand, if oxybutynin helps the wetting improve within a month after treatment begins—which is typical— everyone will feel hopeful. That positive outlook will boost progress all the more.

Choosing Oxybutynin. There are a few *possible* adverse effects associated with oxybutynin, but they can usually be corrected with a lower dose. In fact, because only small doses of the medication are needed to show good results, such reactions are infrequent, occurring perhaps in about 5 percent of children treated.

To understand these reactions, it is helpful to know that oxybutynin reduces the activity of the smooth muscle of the bladder. In rare cases, it may also affect other muscles of the body. Because you may have heard stories about the negative effects of medications, here we present the facts about the most notable ones regarding Ditropan (in order of "occasional" to "no cases reported"):

- **Dry mouth.** This effect, which may accompany a sensation of overheatedness, could cause children to overdrink.
- **Constipation.** Oxybutynin may slow the activity of the colon and contribute to abdominal pain or constipation.
- **Blurry vision.** This is a very unusual adverse effect, caused by an alteration in the function of the eye muscles. If your child does begin taking oxybutynin, you should ask his teachers to tell you if he squints or needs to come closer to the board.
- **Nosebleeds.** In some children, oxybutynin may cause the nose's mucous linings to dry out, resulting in nosebleeds.
- **Crabbiness.** For reasons that are not understood, the medication has been seen to make children "irritable" or act strangely. This effect disappears after the medication is stopped.
- **Asthma.** Oxybutynin may also act on the muscles in the body's airway passages. *Theoretically,* the medication could cause those muscles to contract more strongly and so *theoretically* enhance a child's tendency to be asthmatic. *We have never noted this adverse effect in our practice, and we have never heard of a single case in which it has occurred.* Nevertheless, it is worthwhile to be aware that the possibility exists. Naturally, as with any medication, inform the doctor who is treating your child for asthma about your child's medication for wetting, and follow the doctor's advice.

Please remember that the infrequency with which these effects occur is largely related to the dosing schedule used in the Try for Dry program. Other programs, which may prescribe the dose of

Ditropan by weight—the common method of prescribing medications—are likely to show such side effects more frequently. Our dosing schedule is based not on children's weight but on their age, the extent of their reduced bladder capacity, and their voiding symptoms.

For example, when bedwetting is due to enuresis and children show reduced functional bladder capacity, the Try for Dry approach doses Ditropan as follows:

Age	Dose
5–7 years	Ditropan ¹/₂ tsp. at 8 A.M., 4 P.M., and bedtime
8–12 years	Ditropan ¹/₂ tsp. at 8 A.M. and 4 P.M. and 1 tsp. at bedtime. (For children in this age group who show a *normal* bladder capacity, only give Ditropan 1 tsp. at bedtime.)
12 years and older	Ditropan ¹/₂ tsp. at 8 A.M. and 4 P.M. and 1–2 tsp. at bedtime

These doses may be adjusted by increasing the doses by a half teaspoon (or tablet) every two weeks according to the child's needs (until conventional dose limits are met). Bear in mind that these amounts are given only as an example of what we think would typically be appropriate treatment. Each case is different, however, and must be evaluated individually and thoroughly by your doctor. *Your doctor will determine the dosage for your child and is solely responsible for that determination.*

LARGE BLADDER CAPACITY AND URGE SYNDROME

A small percentage of children wet during the day but stay dry all night. Your answers to the Try for Dry Questionnaire in Chapter 4 and an evaluation by your pediatrician can help you

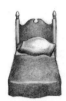

NOT RECOMMENDED:
BLADDER STRETCHING EXERCISES

A commonly prescribed therapy for small bladder capacity is "bladder stretching" exercises (also called retention control training). In such an exercise, when a child feels the need to void, he tries to "hold it" as long as possible. The idea is that strengthening the sphincter muscles, which are responsible for retaining urine, may over time enable the child's bladder to hold more urine.

Although there is some limited medical support for bladder stretching exercises, we have found that the benefits are questionable. First, holding urine in is very hard to do and even can be painful to children. Second, some urologists believe that bladder stretching exercises might be dangerous, because the child could start a long-term habit of tightening the sphincter muscle, which may later cause serious bladder or kidney problems. Third, even if bladder stretching works, the exercises do not help overcome the major cause of bedwetting: deep sleep. Finally, because children who practice the exercises progress so slowly, the results do not justify the time and effort required. If the child works hard at the exercises and still bedwets, he probably will feel even more frustrated than before. As we have seen, success depends on maintaining a positive outlook and building a record of dryness.

rule out other contributors to wetting such as urine infection, incontinence, psychological issues, small bladder capacity, bowel irregularity, and food sensitivities. At least two other conditions may contribute to this *same* pattern of wetting: (1) increased bladder capacity and (2) urge syndrome. In addition to the specific remedies described below for each condition, children may benefit from following a toileting schedule (see "A Voiding Schedule," page 141).

Large Bladder Capacity. If your child has a larger than normal bladder capacity, he may not be emptying his bladder completely when he urinates. (You can measure your child's bladder capacity by following the instructions in Chapter 4.) To help him do so, encourage your child to be patient in the bathroom, so that he empties his bladder. You may even ask him to return to the bathroom and urinate again just a few minutes later. *Note:* Large bladder capacity is not typical of routine bedwetting, so be sure to consult your doctor.

Urge Syndrome. Most children with this problem are between four and nine years old. Their stories are similar: Parents report that their child has always been healthy and dry, but in the past few months, has begun to visit the toilet often and experiences great urgency. If the child doesn't get there in time, she wets. Paradoxically, though, the child either sleeps through the night without wetting or gets up to urinate in the bathroom.

In many children, this increased frequency and urge results from a reduced functional bladder capacity or from an inflammation of the bladder. What causes this inflammation, called nonspecific cystourethritis, is not clear. It seems likely that something "like a viral infection" is behind it.

For example, children tend to get sore throats, and sometimes we find that bacteria cause the soreness, but other times we find no bacterial culprit and conclude that the cause must be a viral infection. Likewise, a child's bladder is prone to inflammation not related to bacteria. But unlike a sore throat, which usually gets better within a week, the bladder may stay inflamed for months without showing signs of improvement. The infection that increased the frequency and urgency and caused the wetting may disappear, but the symptoms persist.

In such cases, the child usually benefits from a sulfa-based antibiotic combined with oxybutynin (to combat small bladder capacity and urgency). If the symptoms still don't improve, you should visit a pediatric urologist.

FREQUENT (OR INFREQUENT) URINATION

In this section, we will address two common conditions in children regarding urination frequency—too frequent daytime voiding and too infrequent daytime voiding—for children who wet only at night and for those who wet only in the daytime.

Remember that unless stated otherwise, you should try our suggested treatments in addition to using the enuresis alarm (for nighttime wetting).

The child who wets only at night.

Too frequently. Children who bedwet commonly urinate more often than normal—throughout the day and night, particularly if their bladder capacity is small. If your child does not wet during the day but does urinate frequently while awake, he may benefit from taking oxybutynin, the same medication used to treat small bladder capacity, during the day. Oxybutynin decreases daytime frequency and eases the urgency to void that your child may feel.

Too seldom. If, however, your child wets only at night and urinates too infrequently—that is, if she urinates less than four times during waking hours—then daytime medication may not be necessary. Setting up a schedule for visiting the bathroom at designated times may be helpful (see "A Voiding Schedule," page 141). Taking a dose of Ditropan before bedtime may also still be helpful, though.

The child who wets only in the daytime.

It is most unusual for a child to wet during the day but not at night. However, because some children do experience such a wetting pattern, we will cover their situation here.

Too frequently. For children who wet only during the day and urinate too often, and for whom incontinence has been ruled out by your doctor, we recommend oxybutynin in addition to the enuresis alarm. Children who wet during the day likely have a reduced bladder capacity.

If you find that this is true of your child (see Chapter 4 for instructions on how to measure bladder capacity), consult your doctor about the possibility of using oxybutynin to help your child learn daytime dryness.

In conjunction with medication and the Happy Bladder Diet (which we present later in this chapter), we recommend that you implement a timed voiding schedule for your child. Also, the child needs to wear the alarm after school during the week and most of the day during weekends as training sessions to "learn" dryness.

Make sure that while at school your child has a small duffel or gym bag with a change of clothes, including dry undergarments and a plastic bag large enough to hold wet clothes. This can be kept in the child's locker or a teacher's closet. Having dry clothes available will save your child from the embarrassment of being sent home, having to wait for you to deliver dry clothes, or, worse yet, being forced to sit in wet clothing until released from class.

Too seldom. If your child indeed has urinary infrequency, wets occasionally during the day, but does not wet at night, her toilet

A VOIDING SCHEDULE

A good way to encourage a child to establish a normal pattern of urination is to set up a schedule. Explain to your child that every day for the next few weeks, you would like her to *try* to urinate every two hours. Whether or not the child "needs" to urinate, she should attempt to do so at the scheduled time. Every time the child tries to void on schedule (even if no urine comes out), reward her by praising her. A few successes should motivate her to keep the schedule.

Here are a few suggestions for making the timed voiding schedule go smoothly:

- For a younger child, say that she will attempt to void on the even hours throughout the day: at 8:00 A.M., 10:00 A.M., 12:00 noon, 2:00 P.M., and so on.
- For a child who is old enough to set an alarm, present him with an inexpensive wristwatch with a timer that can be set to go off every two hours. Medication-reminder timers, which can be set once to sound multiple times throughout the day, are also available through medical supply stores.
- For older children who spend a lot of time on the computer, electronic reminders that pop up periodically may grab their attention.

Whatever you decide, be sure to explain to any adults who may be supervising your child during the day—teachers, coaches, or counselors—that your child must be excused from regular activities and possibly even reminded to use the toilet at the prescribed interval. Remember to make clear to your child that he is not to abuse this privilege by loitering in the halls or using it as an excuse to shirk his academic responsibilities. (We've found that few children actually do misbehave when given this responsibility.)

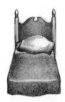

DON'T AVOID FLUIDS

Some children avoid drinking enough fluids through-out the day in a misguided effort to stay dry at night. Going thirsty won't work as the only treatment! In fact, because it can lead to constipation, drinking too little can exacerbate wetting. To help stop wetting, it's much more effective for a child to avoid certain kinds of drinks (such as caffeinated sodas) and refrain from overdrinking.

habits may need improvement. It could be that your child simply "holds off" using the bathroom and wets because her bladder is "overfull." Some children void incompletely because they are too busy to take the time to empty their bladder. They start to void, relieve their sense of pressure, hear a stream of urine, then stop voiding to return to whatever they were engrossed in. Consider trying a timed voiding schedule to encourage her to toilet more frequently. While you are following the voiding schedule, continue recording in the diary (in Chapter 4) the time and amount voided, until the condition improves. Chronic delaying of urination can lead to urinary tract infections, bowel problems, and other bladder complications, so it's important to end such a habit.

To facilitate wetting treatments for a child whose infrequent voiding contributes to day dampness or wetting at school, you may want to write a letter similar to the one below to keep teachers and other adults informed and to ask for their assistance.

Dear [teacher's name],

It has been discovered that [child's name] has enuresis, a condition that results in periodic wetting episodes during the day. As part of our attempt to help [him/her] gain control of [his/her] bladder, we have instituted a timed voiding schedule, which requires that [he/she] attempt to use the toilet every two hours whether or not [he/she] has the urge to go.

To keep it simple, we have instructed [him/her] to ask to be excused from class on even-numbered hours. We would appreciate it if you would see to it that [he/she] is encouraged to leave the room in a manner that is not disruptive to your class and does not draw undue attention to this sensitive issue.

If you have any questions or concerns, you can call me during the day at [phone number] or in the evening at [phone number]. Thank you.

Sincerely,

[your name]

Giggle Wetting. An unusual form of day wetting that occurs when a child laughs, giggle wetting is seen more often in girls than boys, and is infrequent after puberty. The cause of the problem is unknown. In the past, this type of wetting has not responded well to treatment.

Recently, this symptom has been regarded as a result of narcolepsy, a seizure disorder. Just as we have come to understand that for some individuals, staring at a computer screen may trigger a seizure, so laughter can trigger this seizure of wetting. The medication Ritalin is considered the treatment of choice for this seizure disorder. If your child exhibits this kind of wetting, make sure you consult your doctor before choosing to proceed with the program we describe in this book.

OVERPRODUCTION OF URINE AT NIGHT (POLYURIA)

As we explained in Chapter 2, some children who wet by night apparently do so because of a shortage of the antidiuretic hormone (ADH) vasopressin, which is produced in the brain and travels via the bloodstream to the kidneys. A synthetic version of this hormone, called desmopressin or DDAVP, may be prescribed to reduce the volume of urine produced. In many cases, the drug, which is delivered to the bloodstream via a nasal spray, has quickly helped children experience dry nights.

One study published in 1993 reported that DDAVP not only works well in 75 percent of patients, but also that it is particularly effective (91 percent success) in patients with a family history of nocturnal enuresis. Children who wet by night and who also have a genetic predisposition to enuresis, such as having a parent who also wet his or her own bed beyond age six, are likely to respond favorably to desmopressin. For children who bedwet as preteens or older, the use of a small amount of DDAVP as an adjunct to the use of the alarm, Ditropan, the elimination diet, and the bowel program (if needed) adds significantly to the ability to get to dry. This does not seem to be the case in younger children.

For those looking for a quick fix, desmopressin almost fills the bill. However, the drug has a few drawbacks:

1. Not all children who take desmopressin *automatically* get dry: it does not work for everyone. So, before you rely on the medication for an important event, do a "dry run" at home first.

2. When children stop taking the medication, about 80 percent of them show wetting relapses.

3. Physicians have only limited long-term experience with the drug. Because of this, children should not use it for longer than six months.

WHY DRUGS MIGHT "CURE" ENURESIS

The two popular drugs for treating bedwetting, DDAVP and imipramine, both show wetting relapses of about 80 percent after the medication is discontinued. Conversely, they are associated with success for about 20 percent of children. Perhaps the real effect of such medication is to "passively" maintain dryness in the children over the course of a year or so of treatment. Thus when the medication was discontinued, those children who stayed dry may have been really part of the recognized 15 percent spontaneous cure rate for wetting. In other words, the medication remitted the symptom, while "Mother Nature" remitted the problem.

4. One month's supply of desmopressin can be costly for some families. Check your health insurance regarding cost coverage.

5. The drug does not address the likely root problem of bedwetting, which is deep sleep.

6. Desmopressin does not always work, especially during winter cold and flu season, when children are likely to have nasal congestion. When the mucous membranes of the nose are inflamed, the amount of drug absorbed may be insufficient. However, DDAVP is now available in tablet form. This preparation may be opted for children who are congested nasally.

We recommend considering desmopressin if your child fits the correct profile and needs to be dry *on demand* at once. For instance, if she is going away for a special overnight activity or staying with a relative for a short period, the drug may be the best option. However, we do not consider desmopressin to be a

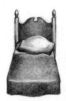

DRINK ENOUGH, BUT NOT TOO MUCH

Obviously, it is better for the child to make less urine at night rather than more. The more urine there is to pass at night, the more times the child will have to get up, and so the more chances for failure and frustration—not to mention interrupted sleep. But it is harmful to withhold liquids completely from a child. Doing so not only may result in constipation, but it does not address the real cause of the problem: deep sleep.

We recommend that children drink in the evening only when they are thirsty—and the parent should decide how much. Ideally, they should drink only the beverages listed in the Happy Bladder Diet (see page 157). Also, they should avoid eating salty or spicy foods, which will only make them thirsty.

good initial treatment to resolve wetting. We recommend that after children use it for the special activity, they should follow the full treatment program (as introduced in Chapter 5) as soon as they return home. We also recommend desmopressin when both parents work and cannot sacrifice a good night's sleep to get up repeatedly in response to an enuresis alarm. For such families, desmopressin may be the best choice, at least for the time being.

Of course, make sure your doctor has evaluated your child before prescribing desmopressin, and be certain that you understand all of the usage instructions.

SUMMARY

On the opposite page is a list of urological symptoms paired with our basic recommendations for treatment. Of course, you need to visit your doctor before proceeding.

THE TRY FOR DRY SONG: VERSE 3

Bladder big, / or bladder small. / The pee in me, / I gotta control.

Refrain
I'm gonna try, / Try for Dry, / and when I do, / I'm gonna be / mighty high!

(See Appendix B for the music and lyrics to the song in its entirety.)

Symptom	Recommendations
Small bladder capacity	Oxybutynin
Large bladder capacity	Encourage child to empty bladder completely when urinating
Urge syndrome	Antibiotic combined with oxybutynin Voiding schedule
Frequent urination	Oxybutynin Voiding schedule
Infrequent urination	Voiding schedule

Remember: Remedies for wetting problems work best in combination. We suggest the enuresis alarm whenever the child and the family can deal with the requirements of alarm use. Similarly, we advise our patients to try to follow the bowel treatment and the elimination diet that appear in the next sections.

Improving Bowel Health

If your child's average bowel movement frequency is less than once a day, try one or more of the following treatments (depending on the severity of the condition):

1. Scheduling daily toileting (below)
2. Changing diet and increasing exercise (page 149)
3. Using a stool softener (page 150)
4. Using a bowel stimulant (page 150)
5. Administering an enema (page 151)

SCHEDULED DAILY TOILETING

Most children who have irregular defecation are able to progress toward regularity by trying to move their bowels *at the same time every morning,* preferably after breakfast. The child should sit on the toilet and attempt to defecate for no more than five minutes: if a movement is coming, it should come in five minutes. Sitting for a longer period just frustrates everybody. Having the child drink a warm beverage (such as hot cocoa) or applying a warmed device to the abdomen (such as a hot water bottle) before he sits on the toilet may help the bowel training process. Also, abdominal massage can help get the bowels going; for a demonstration of proper massage technique, ask a physical therapist.

Some families ask if it is all right for their child to have a daily bowel movement in the afternoon. If your child shows progress toward dryness on schedule, then his personal pattern of defecation may not need to be modified. But our experience suggests that it is worthwhile to make some effort at morning toileting. For one thing, encouraging your child to have a bowel movement before school may itself help relieve stress. Some children feel uncomfortable moving their bowels at school because of sanitary and privacy concerns. Because many children hold in their stool until they come home, and because they tend to be very busy once they are home, the resulting constipation can often complicate treatment of their enuresis (and encopresis, if present).

THE TRY FOR DRY SONG: VERSE 4

It's the poo, / sure enough. / Every morn', / I've gotta do, / doo-doo.

Refrain
I'm gonna try, / Try for Dry, / and when I do, / I'm gonna be / mighty high!

(See Appendix B for the music and lyrics to the song in its entirety.)

DIET AND EXERCISE

We all know by now that eating foods high in fiber is important for good health. And who hasn't heard the call for Americans to add more exercise to their daily lives? Less obvious, however, is the effect that diet and exercise can have on childhood wetting problems. A low-fiber diet can cause constipation, as can a life of inactivity. Is your child getting enough fiber in her diet? Does your child get enough exercise? If not, there are two small changes you can make that could yield very positive results.

More Fiber. Some foods that are high in fiber are bran flakes, apples, peanut butter, whole-wheat bread, and granola bars. Remember to avoid giving your child a heavy load of milk or cheese products, which could lead to constipation. A little applesauce will also promote looser bowels.

More Exercise. Sedentary children may show a tendency to constipation. To maximize your child's chances for success in getting to dry, encourage her to pick a sport or activity and run with it. Whether it's bike riding, swimming, playing soccer, or just the usual childhood horsing around, daily exercise will keep the bowels moving. Minimize couch-sitting and television-watching in your house—not just for the benefit of the child who wets, but for everyone in the family. Schedule a weekly walk in the woods or in the city for kids and parents together. If you lead by example, your child will likely follow.

STOOL SOFTENERS AND STIMULANTS

If you have tried implementing a toileting schedule and changing your child's diet and exercise habits and your child still does not move his bowels daily, or if the bowel movement is dry and hard, consider using an over-the-counter preparation such as mineral oil.

For youths, a common starting dose of mineral oil is one teaspoon to one tablespoon twice a day. Mineral oil, which helps lubricate and soften stools, makes them easier and more comfortable to pass. Mineral oil, though tasteless and odorless, is not very appealing by itself. Most people mix it with orange juice or disguise it by pouring it over pasta. If an excess dose of mineral oil is taken, the extra amount may leak out and stain underwear, so you may need to individualize the dose, such as giving one-half tablespoon of mineral oil twice on one day, then one-half tablespoon once the next day.

You should use such preparations only while the child is learning urinary dryness. Consult your physician if you feel your child requires ongoing use of a stool softener. *Note:* Since some vitamins are fat soluble, do not give your child mineral oil at the same time as a vitamin tablet. Wait about three hours between administering the two. You could also consider giving your child one dose of mineral oil before bedtime, so it will not compete with the absorption of food or vitamins.

Stool Stimulants

If your child does not defecate daily, you should use a natural stimulant such as Senokot. Be mindful that if Senokot induces

THINKING AHEAD

For school-age children, you should initiate a bowel program later in the week, if possible, say, on a Thursday or Friday. If problems such as mineral oil stains, diarrhea, or abdominal cramps develop, they usually take a few days to show up. It's less embarrassing and less distressing for a child if these problems occur at home, not at school. Starting later in the week gives you the whole weekend to resolve them if they come up.

diarrhea, you may need to choose a lower dose of the medication or increase the dosage interval.

ENEMAS

If you suspect your child needs immediate relief from severe constipation—because of difficulty having a bowel movement or because of large, dry stools—consult your doctor about using an enema, such as a pediatric Fleet enema.

To administer an enema, follow these instructions:

1. Place a towel or plastic sheet under the child.
2. Have your child lie on her left side and bring her knees up to her chest.
3. Coat the end of the enema tubing or the tip of the bottle with lubricant and then insert it into the rectum.
4. Let the enema solution flow into the rectum.
5. Ask the child to hold the solution inside for as long as possible.
6. Have the child sit on the toilet to have a bowel movement. Administer one enema per day for two to three days until your child's colon is cleaned out.

When an enema is suggested by your doctor, it is as a last resort. Parents need to be aware that this procedure may be embarrassing and frightening to a child. Before giving an enema, explain to your child why you need to give her an enema and go over the procedure you will be following. Be careful not to be coercive.

If you have never given an enema before, and you are nervous about doing so, ask your doctor if he would supervise this treatment in his office. When we demonstrate the proper technique in our practice, parents are often relieved to see how gentle the procedure is. And children who may have been fearful at first come to accept an enema once they experience its benefit.

ENCOPRESIS

In the medical literature, encopresis is defined as the "repeated passage of feces into inappropriate places (e.g., in clothing or on the floor) whether involuntary or intentional." For our purposes, we will limit our discussion to the involuntary elimination of stool into the underwear. This type of encopresis differs from fecal staining, which commonly results when a child does not wipe himself well enough after defecating.

Most cases of encopresis are associated with constipation accompanied by what we call "overflow incontinence." It can result from a vicious cycle:

1. Children who are constipated may experience pain at defecation and start holding back their stool. The more they withhold their stool, the more constipated they become.

2. When children are fecally impacted, the stool in the colon can become dry and hard as a rock, and the colon becomes large and distended. This distention stretches the linings of the colon so that the muscles and nerves of the colon get stretched

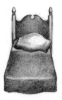

SAMPLE SNACKS

When you're searching for something to satisfy your child at snack time, try one of these treats. Just make sure you read food labels very carefully, and avoid serving food or beverages containing citric acid, artificial colors, or caffeine; dairy products after lunchtime; and snacks with a lot of sugar or salt.

- Crackers with peanut butter
- Bugs on a log: celery sticks filled with peanut butter and topped with raisins
- Crackers
- Raisins
- Fresh fruit or vegetables
- Cereal
- Graham crackers
- Wafers
- Rice cakes
- Roll-ups (such as turkey meat rolled inside a tortilla)
- Nuts
- Sunflower seeds
- Bagel or bagel chips
- Granola bars
- Angel food cake
- Plain donuts
- Popcorn

out, so that the child may have difficulty expelling contained stool (because of weak bowel muscles), lose the sensation of the urge to defecate (perhaps related to poor bowel nerve function), or both.

3. Newly formed stool, which is watery, cannot push its way through the hard, dry stool and consequently the liquid seeps around it and out.

4. The underwear becomes stained with stool that is usually soft and unformed. Thus, parents may mistakenly conclude that their child is not constipated, and do not initiate treatment.

Parents often complain that they do not understand how their child could not smell or feel the stool coming out. The answer is that in addition to the reduced sensation of the stretched bowel, children are so used to the smell of the bowel movements that they become desensitized to it.

In order to treat the encopresis, first the hard stool must be removed, usually with an enema. This initial clean-out is essential. At the same time, the child must begin a regular stool program, including a high-fiber diet, fluids, a stool softener and stimulant, and sufficient exercise. In time, the colon likely will return to its normal size, and normal sensation will resume as defecation becomes regular.

Treating encopresis can take several months; it must be done aggressively and conscientiously to prevent recurring constipation and impaction. Children who are resistant to a regular toilet-sitting program can be motivated with small rewards: say, a nickel or a dime just for sitting on the toilet for five minutes, and two nickels or two dimes if they have a good-sized stool. They can also get rewards (such as a quarter) for self-initiated bowel movements that they make in the toilet at a time other than their regular sitting time.

We also advise that some children older than age five or six be responsible for scrubbing out their own soiled underwear before placing them in the laundry. (A parent should demonstrate how to do it the first time.) Again, stress to your child that this is not intended as a punishment. It is meant to give the child a sense of independence and responsibility, and to increase the child's motivation to defecate in the toilet.

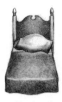

HOLD THE CHEESE

What? No pepperoni pizza for dinner? Yes, your child can eat pepperoni pizza, but *hold the cheese*. This way the child can have his treat and still exclude dairy products from his diet.

For more information about rewarding desired behavior and dealing with undesired behavior, such as a child's refusal to cooperate, see Chapter 7.

Tracking Problem Foods

As we just saw, foods can affect a child's wetting by impairing regular bowel function. Likewise, for years mothers have suspected that certain foods seem to "bother" their children's bladders and bring out wetting tendencies. Just as some people get hives after eating chocolate, get sleepy after sipping a glass of wine, or can't sleep after drinking coffee, some children seem to wet more often after they take in certain foods or beverages. In this section, we will show you how to isolate the problem foods using an elimination diet.

The Happy Bladder Diet is one we've developed in our practice. It's a classic elimination diet, which gets its name from the strategy one takes when trying to isolate a problem food: you *eliminate* the suspected foods and beverages, making sure that your child has none of that type of food while on the diet, and then reintroduce each food or drink one at a time.

Start by withholding for two weeks all of the foods and drinks listed in the left column. Beverages that your child may drink (in moderation) include water, cranberry juice, nectar juice, and apple juice.

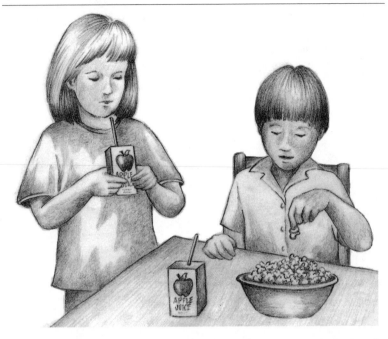

Figure 6-1. The Happy Bladder Diet offers satisfying substitutes for foods and beverages that may be contributing to a child's wetting problem.

After two weeks you may begin reintroducing the "problem" items, one at a time. If wetting occurs after a particular beverage or food is reintroduced, eliminate that item again. You may have found a food or beverage culprit. Then withhold that food or beverage for a few weeks. You may then reintroduce the item and observe your child for any signs that the item is affecting wetting.

WHAT TO DO NEXT

If you find that your child seems to be wetting as a result of consuming any of the beverages or foods listed here, she should refrain from ingesting that substance until wetting has remitted.

THE HAPPY BLADDER DIET

Drinks to Avoid

Satisfying Substitutes

Drinks with carbonation (Pepsi, Coke, 7-Up, and others)
Drinks with caffeine (soda, coffee, tea)

Water

Drinks with artificial colors (Kool-Aid, Hawaiian Punch, Hi-C, and others)
Drinks with citric acid (orange juice, lemon juice, grapefruit juice, and others)

Cranberry juice
Pear or apricot nectar
Apple juice (without added vitamin C)
All-natural, noncitric juices

Milk and other dairy beverages after lunchtime

Milk and other dairy beverages are OK at breakfast and lunch

Foods to Avoid

Satisfying Substitutes

Ice cream after noon

Frozen natural fruit pops (without citric acid and without artificial coloring)

Citrus fruits (oranges, lemons, grapefruit, and others)
Melons (watermelon, cantaloupe, and others)

Apples, pears, bananas, cherries, plums, apricots, nectarines, grapes, raisins, and others

Any pizza with cheese

Pizza with tomato sauce, vegetables, sausage, pepperoni, and other toppings (just hold the cheese)

Sugary foods and candy (such as chocolate bars)

Low-salt popcorn, chips, pretzels, nacho chips (in moderation)
Fresh vegetables with nondairy dip

Vitamin supplements containing artificial colors, vitamin C, or both

Most vitamins without added vitamin C sold at health-food stores

---

THE TRY FOR DRY SONG: FINAL VERSE

It may be. / It may be the milk. / It may be. / It may be the juice. / Or my sweet tooth / on the loose.

Refrain
I'm gonna try, / Try for Dry, / and when I do, / I'm gonna be / mighty high!

(See Appendix B for the music and lyrics to the song in its entirety.)

She can try it from time to time every few months to see if it still causes a problem.

We find that approximately 10 percent of children who wet are being affected by one or more problem foods or drinks listed on page 157. A small percentage of children will become dry just by following the diet and doing nothing else, but the majority benefit from a combination of remedies. In our experience, food sensitivities do not usually single-handedly make a dry child wet, but they can exacerbate existing wetting—and make getting to dry harder.

Summary

In Chapter 5 and in this chapter, we have presented the core of our dryness program: the treatments that you will administer simultaneously to your child, chosen according to his wetting symptoms. In the next chapter, we'll give you a few proven tools that will help you and your child stay on track.

PART THREE

Following Through

Chapter 7

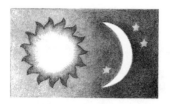

Staying the Course

N OW THAT YOU have chosen the remedies that suit your child's wetting behavior, let's consider the best ways to ensure your child's success. We have learned that there are three essential ingredients in any permanent dryness plan: (1) motivation, (2) reinforcement, and (3) responsibility. In this chapter, we present a number of methods that you can use to bolster your child's efforts. Rewarding your child for engaging in desired behaviors, such as putting on the enuresis alarm without being reminded or changing wet sheets, will help her build good habits and make more and more progress. As we discuss in the second part of this chapter, the right incentive—ranging from praise to extra privileges to a material object—can work wonders on your child's motivation to keep trying.

Motivation

Does your child want to get dry? If so, why? Perhaps she is missing out on sleepovers and has decided to focus on solving this problem once and for all. Or maybe she's just tired of waking up wet. Perhaps a younger sibling has already gotten dry easily. Children express many reasons for starting the dryness program, but they all boil down to this: "I want control over my body." A child who is motivated by a feeling of ownership of the problem is already ahead of the game. So it is very important for parents to explain /that although the child is not to blame for wetting, since it is usually beyond her control, the child is responsible for doing the work necessary to stop wetting. However, there is no need to overburden your child; help her focus not only on her daily tasks, but also on the wonderful sense of pride she will feel when she finally overcomes her wetting.

Reinforcement

One of the most difficult challenges for children undergoing treatment for wetting is merely sticking with a program. When progress is slow, when wetting shows no signs of remitting, children can lose heart and ask to stop treatment. On the other hand, when a child has made a great deal of progress but has not quite reached his goal, he may get impatient and want to quit. You, as the parent, need to be prepared to help your child overcome the doubts, the tedium, and the frustration that will come with treatment. In this section we'll explore the issue of reinforcement: giving rewards and other affirmative feedback in order to help kids stay on track.

THE STAR CHART

You will find that one of the most useful tools at your disposal is a star chart, like the one shown in Figure 7-1. The chart is a good way to reward a child for approximating and accomplishing dry nights. The chart also functions as a dryness calendar—that is, a

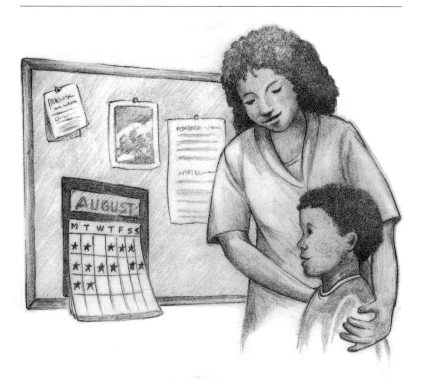

Figure 7-1. The star chart, or dryness calendar

record of your child's dry days and nights, so that he knows when and how to taper use of the alarm and when he has reached his goal of fourteen consecutive dry days and nights. (See "Tapering Treatments and Beyond," page 175.)

When used in conjunction with the enuresis alarm, this chart is very effective. First, help your child fill in the days of the week and their corresponding dates. Then, every night that your child wears the alarm, he should put the letter *A* or a check mark in the appropriate space on the chart. By marking the chart himself, your child is not only monitoring his compliance with the pro-

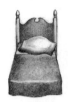

CONSISTENCY COUNTS

In our practice, children with enuresis (that is, those who have no structural problem in their urinary system) remain wet when they *inconsistently* follow the combined treatment program—despite trying the alarm, medication, dietary changes, and a bowel regimen. Especially if the child does not wear the alarm as instructed, little progress should be expected. If, however, the child wears the alarm as scheduled every night for a month—dutifully recording her compliance on the chart—but is making no progress despite being awakened by the parents, a further medical examination is recommended.

gram, he is also reminding himself to wear the alarm the next night.

Decide with your child where in the house to place the progress chart. Many children are sensitive about their wetting and may prefer the chart to be in their own room, where it is not visible to everyone who comes into your home. Others may be eager to show their progress to all who are interested and will be perfectly happy to have it proudly displayed on the kitchen refrigerator. In any case, make sure it is easily accessible and very noticeable to the child.

The child should get a gold star on the progress calendar for every night he stays dry all night; he should get a silver star when he wet but only enough to dampen his underpants before getting to the toilet in time to finish the void. Silver stars indicate that the child is making progress but needs to get up more quickly to urinate. The child should receive no star after a wet night. Instead he should write the letter *W* on the chart.

There are a variety of stickers available in card shops and novelty stores with various motifs that a younger child may enjoy.

Shop around and make the experience a way to get the child excited about the program. Since stars or stickers may feel baby-ish to older children, let them devise their own system of record-keeping. Some children may respond to decorative rubber stamps or, depending on their age, may draw their own progress chart or create one on a computer. A handmade chart or calendar that is meaningful to the child may have a positive influence on his success. This is a time to have fun and be creative.

If you are consulting a health-care professional, bring the chart with you to every visit. It will be a graphic aid in helping your doctor see your child's progress, and the doctor can praise your child and recognize his efforts.

ADDITIONAL REINFORCERS

Some professionals suggest that rewards beyond the star chart or progress calendar are not necessary, because nobody is more motivated to get dry than the wet child. Peculiarly enough, this is not always true. Young children are generally easily motivated by the star chart and quite often do not require additional rein-forcers, but sometimes older children, on the other hand, are absolutely convinced that they cannot be helped and have re-signed themselves to their "fate." They may say, "It's no big deal. I can handle it," or, "It's really not that bad." Other chil-dren may be afraid to try something new or may lack the self-confidence to get going on their own and aggressively take charge of the situation. And if an enuretic child has been teased by sib-lings or embarrassed in front of peers, he may fear that a treat-ment program would attract added attention and cause further humiliation. This is particularly true of older enuretic children.

Sometimes the only way to break through a wall of denial or hopelessness is a good reward. You must choose a reward that is age-appropriate and desirable to your child. Just like adults, individual children have very different tastes: one child's reward may be completely unappealing to another child. Rewards do not have to be material. Some of the best rewards are spending time with the parent doing something special together, such as playing a game of the child's choice, baking, playing sports, making an art project, and so on. Some children might want to earn points that can be traded for privileges or other rewards.

Children need immediate rewards to change behavior. You can reward compliance with the program, dryness, or both. Children who are noncompliant can often be motivated with minimal nightly rewards for simply using the alarm appropriately, as well as taking responsibility for wet sheets and clothes. (But you should also try to find out why they don't comply. They may be thinking, "If I do this program but stay wet, I'll feel even worse about myself . . . so I just won't do it.") An extra sticker on their chart, a baseball card, sugarless bubble gum, or a small amount of money can do the trick.

If your child is compliant but is losing interest in the program or getting frustrated that she is not becoming dry as quickly as expected, you can recharge her motivation by rewarding dry nights. Start by rewarding a single dry night, then two dry nights, then four, and so on. When the wetting has fully remitted (according to our schedule), an additional reward might be appropriate.

Be careful not to make the material reward the object of the program. Getting dry is the objective, not a new video game or a trip to an amusement park. Never withhold or threaten to withhold rewards that are promised or owed as part of this program because the child has broken another family rule. Doing so undermines the child's motivation to comply. Isolate this reward program from any other type of incentive system in which your child participates. For example, if you agreed to let the child choose what video the family will rent on Saturday if he remained dry for five nights this week, do not threaten to take away that privilege because he did not do his homework. If he accomplishes the agreed-upon goal, he should get his promised reward. Similarly, do not allow your child to earn a video for doing his homework if the video is the reward for staying dry. If he knows he can earn the desired video by doing his homework, this will minimize the value of the incentive to stay dry.

We do not recommend that you give additional rewards to children who already show that they are internally motivated: in such cases, adding an extra reward may weaken a child's own internal desire to succeed.

REWARDING DAYTIME DRYNESS

Reinforcement programs also offer great incentive for daytime wetters to get dry. We usually target two desired behaviors for daytime wetters: (1) staying dry during a specific interval of time, and (2) urinating in the toilet.

The choice of an appropriate targeted time interval depends on the frequency of the child's wetting. For instance, children who wet only once a day can be rewarded for staying dry all day. Children who wet five times a day may need more frequent rewards, say, initially for every two-hour time period that they remain dry. Then extend it to four hours, then six, then eight, and so on until the child remains dry all day.

In addition to rewarding dryness, it is important to increase the child's frequency of using the toilet. Therefore, you can reward your child with a small treat, such as sugarless bubble gum, each time she urinates in the toilet. In this way, eventually you will change the undesirable behaviors of wetting and not using the toilet to the desirable alternatives.

Many parents consider rewards to be bribes. They feel that the child should not have to be rewarded for something expected of him. In our view, a bribe is an incentive given to someone for doing something wrong, while a reward is an incentive given to someone for doing something right. After all, that's how our society operates. In addition, bribes are given as an inducement, before the desired behavior occurs; rewards are given only after the desired behavior has occurred.

Responsibility

It is a good idea to review periodically with your child his responsibilities regarding the dryness program, such as:

1. Wearing the alarm as required
2. Changing his own wet nightclothes and sheets (with your help)
3. Filling in the progress calendar

Sit down with your child and make a formal list of tasks that she is expected to complete, similar to the one provided below. Remember, by giving the child the opportunity to approve her list, you can be sure that the child does not perceive these tasks as punishments.

I, _____, agree to be responsible for doing the following things:

1. _____
2. _____
3. _____

_____   _____
Child's signature   Date

_____   _____
Parent's signature   Date

Remember that we specifically recommend against humiliating or blaming children in any way for their wetting. Shaming a child can cause psychological harm far worse than the enuresis alone. Children of any age, however, can be encouraged to take responsibility for their treatment. Explain to your child that part of getting dry requires that he do everything he can to help himself. Some younger children may need help understanding that parents cannot magically solve all problems. Remind the child that you and others involved in his care have provided the self-help tools he needs to become dry, namely, the methods presented in this book. Also, assure him that you will be there to help and to make sure he knows what to do and when.

WHOSE JOB IS IT, ANYWAY?

The issue of taking responsibility for one's wetting problem surfaces in the question of clean-up. Who should be the one to take care of the wet sheets and pajamas at night, and launder the wet bedding and nightclothes? The parent or the child or both?

Our answer depends on your situation and your perception of your child's readiness for such tasks. The child, if capable, should at least strip the wet bed, rinse out wet underwear, and replace the alarm on clean underwear before returning to bed. If the child is old enough, physically capable, and does not take an inordinate amount of time doing so (so as not to lose sleep needed for school), she should be responsible for remaking the bed, too. Younger children may need some help, but older children should accept as much of the responsibility as they can handle. Teenagers, for example, could even wash their own soiled laundry in the washing machine the next day. Of course, if your child is still too deeply asleep at night to complete these tasks, you may want to save some of the clean-up for the child to do in the morning.

BEYOND THE ORDINARY

"The reward program worked, but just for a week. We need something to keep her interested longer."

Many parents see instant success after they begin the reward program. In just a few days of treatment with the alarm and perhaps a medication, a child motivated by sparkling stickers or special treats may achieve new dryness. Most children, like adults, lose interest in the reward if they have gotten it several times. Therefore, it is important to alternate rewards to maintain the child's motivation when the parent senses that the child is habituating to the previously given reward. Talking to the child about what he would like to earn as a reward is likely to give you many suitable alternatives.

One successful approach recognizes that sometimes the joy comes from getting something unexpected. So when the usual rewards seem to lose their appeal, set up a prize bowl. Buy a variety of inexpensive treats, wrap them in bright-colored paper, and put them in a small glass bowl or fishbowl. The child can reach into the bowl and pull out a "surprise" treat when he has attained his goal. For some kids, the anticipation of reaching into the bowl motivates them much more than receiving a predictable reward.

Children can be told, in a neutral manner, that after wetting they should gather their soiled garments and bedding and take them to a designated place, such as a hamper or laundry room. Performing such tasks can help teach them to assume control of their own problem. Children are more likely to get to dry when they see themselves as the person in charge of the mission.

Clean-up chores should never be forced on a child as a punishment for wetting. Some misguided parents blame their child for wetting intentionally, and believe that making the child handle his own mess will deter him from wetting again. In fact, laying more guilt on an already stressed-out child may actually worsen the wetting. The parents end up launching a vicious cycle: wetting episodes elicit shameful feelings in the child, and the parents' negative reaction exacerbates the problem.

We believe that children wet not because they want to be wet, but because they have not yet learned how to stay dry. Of course, parents should share the burdens of the wetting program—such as getting up when they hear the alarm (since many children do not hear it) and getting the child out of bed and into the bathroom as soon as the alarm sounds. Parents must also assume responsibility for administering praise and rewards (stars, stickers, and so on) promptly and faithfully. With this view in mind, it is appropriate to expect a child to help with the clean-up chores, along with the other components of our program.

As with other aspects of our program, we rely on you, the parent, to know what is best for your individual child. As long as your child is making progress to dryness and you are not acting in a punitive manner, you should be confident in your decisions about household tasks.

Summary

As we have indicated, everyone in the family benefits if the enuretic child becomes dry. It is extremely helpful if siblings cooperate or at the very least refrain from making the situation more stressful. The main objective is to create an environment in which everyone does his or her part for the common good during the eight to twelve weeks of the program.

When setting up a reward system, do not promise more than you can deliver. Children often have big ideas about what they want, and parents are often anxious to please their children. Rather than promise a large reward, such as a new bike, for staying dry for two months, it is better to start by rewarding small successes, because children need immediate reinforcement.

Help your child set and achieve realistic goals. Although achieving what you set out to do is often more rewarding than the reward itself, rewards become the proof that the goal has been accomplished.

Finally, remember that the praise and approval of a parent is the best reward any child can receive. Give that reward often, for every dry night and for all of his efforts to comply with the program.

Chapter 8

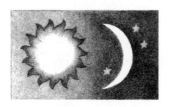

Finishing Up

IN THIS CHAPTER, we describe the progress of a typical child through the treatment program. In this example, the child's situation is as follows:

1. The child has nightly bedwetting due to primary nocturnal enuresis. The child exhibits regular bowel habits.
2. The chosen treatments are an enuresis alarm (for deep sleep), oxybutynin (for reduced bladder capacity), calendar stickers to reward night dryness, and an elimination diet to guard against the possibility that foods or beverages may impair the treatment process.

Then we move on to the final phase of the program, tapering. You will learn when to start gradually discontinuing use of the alarm and the other treatments you have chosen.

Typical Progress to Dryness

The following timetable, based on our clinical experience, is an estimate of the progress toward dryness that a typical child shows. Each child progresses at his or her own pace: some children may react with a few dry nights almost immediately, while others may take a few weeks before they begin to show improvement. If your child shows improved dryness only slowly at first, please remain optimistic in the face of her understandable frustration. Express your confidence that if she stays with the program, improvement will come. (For effective ways of overcoming the hurdles that many children and families face during the getting-to-dry process, see Chapter 9.)

AFTER TWO WEEKS

After two weeks of treatment, you may find that wetting still happens every night, but the volume of urine excreted has decreased. Or, you may find that whereas the wetting used to happen three times nightly, now it occurs only once or twice a night.

At this point it is fair to begin to reintroduce, one at a time, foods or beverages that were restricted. If after you reintroduce such foods your child shows no increase in wetting, then your child is probably one of the 90 percent of children with enuresis who do not show food sensitivity. Go ahead and keep gradually reintroducing the food products that were eliminated. On the other hand, if you give your child soda in the evening and then her wetting increases, you may suspect that soda could be offending a "sensitive" bladder. So restrict soda again for a few more weeks, to give the child a chance to show further improvement.

AFTER ONE MONTH

At this time a child who had been wet nightly (several times a night) should have had two to three nights of near dryness and one to two nights of complete dryness in the previous two weeks. On the remaining nights of the previous two weeks, the child was wet, but not drenched, and wet fewer times per night than before.

If you have seen little progress by now, don't worry. However, you should contact your doctor to see if your child needs a slightly higher dose of medicine. Also, perhaps your child has less than normal bowel regularity that was not discovered earlier. Or your youngster may be sneaking foods and drinks off of the diet. Otherwise, continue what you are doing. Be sure the alarm sensor pads are sewn on in a good location in the underwear, where they will be moistened should wetting happen.

AFTER TWO MONTHS

After the second month, you should have seen further progress in dryness in comparison with the one-month interval. The exact number of dry days and nights varies with each child, but you should feel that your child is on his way to fourteen consecutive dry days and nights by the third month.

AFTER THREE MONTHS

By now your child should have attained or be very close to attaining a remission in wetting: fourteen *consecutive* dry days and nights. Once you have reached this goal, it's time to begin gradually tapering the treatment program.

Tapering Treatments and Beyond

After your child's wetting has remitted, you likely will see more clearly how the wetting problem was caused by some combination of deep sleep, small bladder size, diet sensitivities, and bowel elimination problems. Though each of these factors may arise

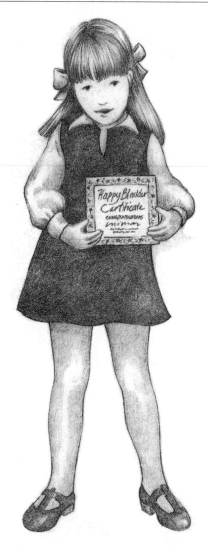

Figure 8-1. A certificate of achievement celebrates success and helps reinforce a child's desire to stay dry.

from a physiological difficulty, your child "learned" to be dry: he was trained to sense an impending bladder contraction and then inhibit it.

For the effects of this learning process to be long-lasting, treatment should be gradually phased out, or tapered, rather than stopped abruptly. Just as a child who fractures her leg wears a cast for a few weeks, your child "healed" her wetting problem with the help of a specific therapeutic device, namely, this dryness program. However, a child with a newly healed fracture only gradually goes from walking with crutches to walking with a cane, to walking unassisted, to running. Likewise, even though your child's wetting has now stopped, she needs to gradually resume her normal bedtime routine.

Based on our experience, we have devised a preferred order in which treatments should be tapered:

Step 1. Phase out the use of the alarm. (See the alarm schedule in Chapter 5 for details on how to do so.)

Step 2. Phase out using the medication.

Step 3. Phase out the bowel program, assuming that your child still moves her bowels daily.

Step 4. Gradually reintroduce any foods or beverages that you found contributed to your child's wetting.

Let's take these one at a time. During any of the following phaseouts, if your child has two or more wet nights over a two-week period, go back to full treatment. After your child gets to dry again, try once more to taper the treatments. If the wetting relapses a second time, consult your doctor.

PHASING OUT THE ALARM

As the primary tool in getting so many children to dry, the use of the enuresis alarm must not be haphazardly or abruptly dis-

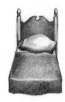

EARNING A CERTIFICATE

Once your child has achieved fourteen consecutive dry days and nights, make a special certificate commemorating the achievement. Have your doctor sign and date it. You can even hold a ceremony celebrating your child's achievement, which will help reinforce his or her desire to stay dry. In addition, we can send you a "Happy Bladder Certificate of Dryness" suitable for framing. Some children we know have proudly displayed their certificates of dryness, even though they were very secretive when they were still wetting. If you'd like to receive a Happy Bladder Certificate, just write to us at the following Internet address:

http://www.tryfordry.com

continued. It is important to carefully phase it out according to the five-step schedule of proven success that we presented in Chapter 5. For details, see "The Alarm Schedule," pages 113–115.

PHASING OUT THE MEDICATION

Make sure that you consult the doctor who prescribed the medication regarding its tapering.

A common schedule for phasing out medicine that has been taken three times daily is the following:

Step 1. Give your child the afternoon and evening doses of the medication for one week.

Step 2. If wetting does not relapse by the end of that week, then give your child only the evening dose of the medication every night for one week.

Step 3. If wetting does not relapse, then give the evening dose every other night for one week.

Step 4. If there is no relapse of wetting, give one dose on two nights of one week.

Step 5. If there is no relapse of wetting, give one dose on one night of one week.

Step 6. If there is no relapse of wetting, discontinue using the medication. If wetting occurs on more than one night of the week, go back to the previous step and try again.

PHASING OUT THE BOWEL REGIMEN

As you will recall, the bowel program involves the use of a daily toileting schedule, a bowel stimulant, and a stool softener, alone or in combination. Though you should discontinue the use of stool softeners and bowel stimulants according to the following guidelines, it is a good idea to stick to the schedule of daily toileting. Many families happily find that after stopping the bowel program, their children continue the good habit of regular bowel movements.

Step 1. Phase out the use of the bowel stimulant (such as Senokot), if you were using one, over two weeks.

Step 2. If the bowels remain regular, phase out the use of the stool softener (such as mineral oil), if you were using one, over the next two weeks.

If, while working toward dryness, your child cannot have daily bowel movements without the bowel program, then have her stay on the program until she does.

PHASING OUT THE ELIMINATION DIET

If you have withdrawn a particular food from your child's diet because you found that it was contributing to wetting, now is the time to gradually reintroduce that food.

If more than one food caused problems, try returning one food at a time to your child's diet. Wait a few days, and if there seems to be no reaction, reintroduce the next food.

If persistent wetting occurs when your child has a particular food or beverage, he should probably eat or drink that food or beverage only on special occasions when it will not matter if he has a wetting episode.

Keep in mind, though, that food sensitivities are by no means consistent or pervasive. A drink that seems to cause wetting one night may have no effect another night. Such mechanisms are often unpredictable. (Even otherwise continent adults occasionally wet the bed after drinking an alcoholic beverage.) And remember that only about 10 percent of children who wet seem to have any kind of food problem that contributes to the wetting.

Is Wetting Cured Forever?

Our dryness program—using an enuresis alarm, taking medication if appropriate, following a bowel regimen, and avoiding problem foods—works by removing the *symptom* of wetting. But the program does not cure the root problem in so many cases: deep sleep. No long-term studies have been done to predict if wetting will someday return in adolescence, young adulthood, middle age, or older age. We do know anecdotally that for some adults, wetting may reappear in the midst of stressful situations (during college exam periods, personal relationship problems, alcohol use, service in the armed forces).

We use the following phrases to describe the stages of dryness:

- **Remission of wetting:** fourteen consecutive dry days and nights within four months of the beginning of the enuresis treatment plan
- **Continued success with remission:** no relapse for six months after enuresis treatment has been discontinued

• **Complete success with remission:** continued dryness for two years after treatment has been discontinued

About 15 percent of children with primary nocturnal enuresis whose wetting has remitted in response to our program will relapse within one year. This is a much lower relapse rate than for other treatments (such as taking imipramine or DDAVP by itself, which has a relapse rate of about 80 percent). If your child has more than two episodes of wetting by day or night in any given month after you have tapered treatments, your child has relapsed. After the family doctor has reaffirmed that incontinence is unlikely and determined that your child has no urine infection, you should begin the dryness program again.

First, remeasure the functional bladder capacity (see "Measuring Bladder Capacity and Urinary Frequency," page 75) to find out whether it has returned to pretreatment values or has indeed increased. If it has increased, go ahead and follow the original treatment program again. If functional bladder capacity is still at pretreatment values or if this is a second relapse, consult your doctor.

Usually, children who have relapsed eventually do get dry again. In children who have had several relapses, a medical examination may reveal the cause. (See Appendix C for the most common disorders that lead to incontinence.)

The Possibility of Incontinence

We know that our treatment plans are effective in children with enuresis. If the wetting does not remit or at least improve after one month of treatment, and compliance with the program has been good, we then must consider the possibility that wetting actually relates to incontinence. Remember that we define incontinence as wetting that results from abnormalities in the urinary tract. After one month of treatment with little progress, you have three choices, which you should consider in consultation with your doctor:

1. Continue to use the dryness program for another two months, making adjustments in the use of the enuresis alarm, the medication, the bowel program, the diet, and other treatments. (See Chapter 9 for details.)
2. Switch to another program, perhaps a medication-only approach such as DDAVP. (See Chapter 6 for more details.)
3. Seek the advice of a pediatric urologist. (See Appendixes C and D.)

Didn't Get to Dry?

The most common reason for wetting to persist despite treatment is that compliance with the program was unsatisfactory. Perhaps the alarm was used inconsistently, or the child would not allow you to observe his stooling habits, or you just couldn't stop your child from sneaking problem foods.

The first step in improving your child's cooperation in the program is to talk it over with her. Try to find out why she does not follow a program that could help her and improve her self-image. Noncompliance may be a sign of other problems. If your child also resists doing other activities (such as homework and household chores), or really does not want to be dry, it is best to resolve these issues before starting the program again. It is often helpful to consult with a behavior therapist or pediatric psychologist who is familiar with dryness programs and skilled at handling noncompliance with medical treatments.

Summary

If all goes well, roughly ten weeks after your child became dry, each of the treatments will have been phased out. (The bowel program may involve an extra two weeks.) If, on the other hand, you run into any obstacles along the way, you will want to turn to the next chapter, which offers solutions to a variety of common problems encountered on the path to dryness.

CHAPTER 9

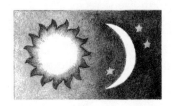

A Troubleshooting Guide

IN THE PRACTICE of medicine, the key to curing a person is properly matching the treatment to needs of the individual. This is especially true when it comes to wetting in children. In a sense, the easy part is determining the causes of wetting. The hard part is selecting and fine-tuning the appropriate treatments to suit a given family's circumstances. (Although we have written this book as a self-help guide, you may want to consult your family doctor or health professional to find the combination of treatments that best fit your family.)

For example, a family distracted by divorce, a recent death, or a sudden move may be better off waiting until the problems settle, or pursuing a passive treatment that does not require their active participation (such as DDAVP). Another family, whose members cannot expend their energy on laundry, may need to permit the child to wear the alarm attached to cloth underwear underneath disposable training pants.

In this chapter, we present many real examples of families with special needs. In our clinical practice, we have seen children and families with specific situations that may complicate getting to dry. These clinical situations are not uncommon, so we will single them out here. However, every child is special, and each family member brings a unique perspective and set of needs to the table.

Many parents are already so frustrated by their child's wetting that they have decided: "I'm not going to bother anymore!"

> *"Why should I follow the advice in this book? My kid still wets even though I have exhausted my pediatrician, my friends . . . I tried having my child fast from liquids after dinner, the bell, even punishment. What makes you think you can get my child dry when everything else has failed?"*

Families who have tried to treat wetting before reading this book may find the most common treatments we use familiar. In fact, they are likely to be the *same* treatments that the family has already tried. The likely reason the treatments have failed is because they were not followed correctly. The cases presented in this chapter will help you perform the treatment procedures faithfully, and ensure that your child has a good chance of reaching dryness.

Concerns about the Enuresis Alarm

Sporadic rather than consistent use of the alarm is one of the most common reasons for treatment failure. If the child does not wear the alarm consistently, he will not learn how to become dry.

Some children remove the alarm from its pocket during sleep. To guard against this, check that the sensor is correctly positioned while your child is asleep, before you go to bed. If necessary, attach adhesive tape over the wire onto the outside of the child's underpants. This will make the alarm sensor more difficult to remove.

If the sensor is too far from the site of first urination, it will not sound at the time of wetting. Experiment with the placement of the sensor pocket: put it higher on the underwear for boys and lower for girls. Also, if your child tends to sleep to one side, the pocket may need to be sewn off-center.

"The alarm wakes us up, but by the time we get to my son's room, the bed is already wet."

The alarm will be effective only if a parent responds to it promptly, in other words, before *all* the urine in the bladder has come out. If you and your spouse both sleep heavily, one of you will need either to sleep closer to your child—by, say, moving him temporarily to a room closer to yours—or to amplify the sound of the alarm with a portable intercom, such as a nursery monitor. Also, make sure that you are not going to bed overtired. Your child could also need a larger dose of oxybutynin to help "slow" bladder emptying during sleep.

"The alarm went off the way it was supposed to, but it didn't wake my daughter up. It would blare for hours. We got tired of hearing it, so we stopped using it."

Remember that you or your spouse, *not* your child, will most likely be the ones initially to respond to the alarm. Reread the alarm instructions in Chapter 5 if you need more details.

"Is it OK for my six-year-old to sleep in disposable training pants (such as Pull-Ups) while wearing the alarm?"

There are conflicting opinions on this issue. Some professionals believe that using disposable training pants sends the child mixed messages: "It's OK to wet as long as you are wearing a Pull-Up," or, "We want you to stay dry during the night and urinate into the toilet." Also, some say that disposable training pants infantilize a child.

Our advice: Use your own judgment regarding disposable training pants, but remember that if your child makes little or no progress toward dryness while wearing training pants, you should refrain from using them.

> *"My wife and I both work full-time, and we need our rest. We just can't get up many times a night and then manage to be productive the next day. Plus, our son sleeps in the same room with his older brother. So no one in the family will get enough sleep with that alarm in the house."*

If you and your family feel strongly that the enuresis alarm will be too disruptive, you may want to consider treating the wetting initially with desmopressin. Although this hormone may work effectively, the relapse rate, once treatment is stopped, is high. You could start with the hormone therapy and use it until your schedules permit the time and flexibility you need to carry out the alarm treatment (perhaps in the summertime, for example).

> *"I can't use the alarm, because when my mother tells me to go to bed, I fight with my sheets and pillow to get to sleep. The alarm gets in the way, so I pull it off."*

In such cases parents should consider placing the alarm on the child's underwear after the "fighter" has gotten to sleep.

> *"There's no arguing with him: my child just will not use the alarm."*

If your child absolutely refuses to cooperate and wear the alarm, first, talk with your child about it. Some children are embarrassed and worried that they will be teased by siblings or others. Some children do not want to get up in the middle of the night. If your child's opposition to using the alarm is part of a series of power struggles between you and your child, consult a mental health professional before attempting to treat the enuresis. Trying to force a child to participate in a program with as many demands as this one is a setup for failure.

Some children will not use the alarm because they are afraid of it. One diplomatic approach is to meet your child halfway. Instead of *wearing* the buzzer, perhaps your child will agree to put it under the bed. Doing so could raise his awareness of wetting just enough to facilitate dryness. See also the suggestions in "Introducing the Alarm to Your Child," page 112.

If you decide that alarm use is out of the question for now, try to follow the other components of the program. In addition to these, consider carrying your child to the toilet at timed intervals during the night (see "Scheduled Lifting: An Alternative Approach," pages 116–117). Also, try to build mental cues on controlling night dryness by talking to the child about responding to her bladder urges. Have the child keep a record of wet and dry nights to reinforce her achievements. Though not an ideal approach, these techniques will keep you working toward a positive conclusion. Perhaps after some initial successes, your child will change her mind and agree to wear the alarm.

Concerns about Medication

OXYBUTYNIN

The dose of oxybutynin in our approach is based on your child's functional bladder capacity (as you measured it in Chapter 4), your child's age, and your child's response to the medication. If your child does not attain dryness within the time periods outlined in Chapter 8 (see "Typical Progress to Dryness," page 174), then your doctor may want to increase the dosage. Usually the dose is raised gradually, at three-day intervals in half-teaspoon or half-tablet amounts. Your doctor can give you more details. Always talk to your doctor about changing dosages; never do so on your own.

As we mentioned before, one helpful indicator that oxybutynin is working is red cheeks. In many children, if wetting has not improved and the child's cheeks are not flushed, the child may need a higher dose of medication.

"I stopped giving my son the oxybutynin medication because we finished the bottle."

Some parents may misunderstand the dosing of oxybutynin and assume that when the medication in the bottle is gone, they should stop giving it. To the contrary: continue giving the medication according to your doctor's prescription. If the medication runs out, call the doctor for a refill. Most children need the medication until dryness is attained, commonly for three months of treatment and then for a few weeks during tapering.

"My daughter got to dry by taking DDAVP, but then she started wetting again even though she was still taking the medication."

One common cause of relapses in children who are taking DDAVP is a cold or a sinus infection. These conditions increase nasal congestion, which, as we explained in Chapter 6, impairs the body's ability to absorb the DDAVP. You can consult your doctor to treat the congestion or, if you think it's just a cold, wait until it passes before restarting the medication.

Another consideration is that if a teenager is responsible for administering the "spray" himself, he may not know when to stop using the bottle. Each bottle contains a certain maximum number of puffs. Beyond that number, even if the bottle still has some liquid inside, it will deliver too little medication with each puff. So in effect, the child has stopped getting the hormone, and the wetting will relapse. So make sure you explain the dosage system to your child, and supervise him carefully. Also, consider using the newly available tablet preparation of the drug.

Concerns about Bowel Habits

"I can't get my son to go poo every day."

Consult your doctor about this issue. If the family—especially your child—is committed to following the treatment plan, bowel regularity usually does improve.

Concerns about Diet

"We really followed the elimination diet, but withholding the foods I suspected never produced results."

If you've seen no benefit from the elimination diet, it's possible that no foods exacerbate your child's wetting. But remember, it's worth the effort to double-check on your child's compliance with the diet. You may have assumed that your child was following the diet all day long when in fact he was spending all of his lunch money on soda and enjoying an unrestricted diet at friends' houses. Ask your child to be truthful with you about it. Explain the reasoning behind the diet, and make sure he wants to try the program. Noncompliance with the diet may reflect noncompliance with other aspects of the treatment plan as well. So, go over each part of the treatment program again, and clearly lay out what your child's responsibilities in the program will be (see "Responsibility," page 168). Perhaps you can also work out a reward system, so that your child can see the short-term benefit of sticking to the diet.

Other Concerns

Although we cannot hope to speak to every difficulty you may have while following our program, we would like to address what we have found to be the most common problems that families encounter.

THE FOLLOWING is an excerpt from a message posted on the Internet:

> My son is just 5, and has been out of diapers since age 3½. The problem is that he can't keep his pants dry. . . . We have tried everything: bribery, contests, begging, pleading, even anger. . . . We have also tried to ignore it, hoping that it'll go away. Well, now he starts kindergarten in September and I am so worried that this problem won't be resolved by then. He wets the bed at night, but I am not concerned by that as much as I am by the daytime wetting. Any suggestions?

Many preschools require every student to be toilet trained. As enrollment time approaches, parents tend to become anxious about their child's toilet training, which can lead them to put undue pressure on the child. Be careful: children may respond to their parents' surge in anxiety by simply refusing to cooperate.

If you can find a quality preschool that does not have this requirement, you and your child will be more relaxed about toilet training—and probably more successful. Many children become trained soon after beginning preschool, because they have regular trips to the bathroom, where they try to use the toilet and where they see their peers using the toilet. (Children often respond to this "peer pressure" from older siblings, too.)

If, however, your only choice is a preschool that requires a potty-trained child, try to work at training by making it rewarding for the child. First, be sure that your child is developmentally ready for potty training by noting when your child can (1) walk to the toilet, (2) lower and raise her own underwear, and (3) tell you when she is "peeing" or "pooping."

Once you have decided to begin training, make sure the child has a comfortable potty chair that lets her feet touch the floor—for leverage and for a feeling of security. The child can decorate the potty chair with stickers, either before training begins or after she has earned them for successes. Bring the child to the potty chair every couple of hours in a relaxed, noncoercive manner. Each time the child successfully uses the potty, you should give her a reward and moderate praise—profuse praise may scare or put too much pressure on your child. Children who are resistant or afraid to sit on the potty chair need a small reward and praise just for sitting on the potty and trying to urinate or have a bowel movement.

If your child is clearly not ready to be trained, you are better off not engaging in a power struggle over the issue. If you take a few months off from training, but leave the potty chair out, and refrain from nagging or criticizing your child about not using the potty, she will probably be successful the next time around.

Although developmentally delayed children are likely to lag in potty training, just because your child is not potty trained at age three does not mean that your child is delayed. Try to resist the influence of well-meaning grandparents or family friends, who may brag to you that another child was dry at night and during

CHILDREN WITH SPECIAL NEEDS

Children with developmental delays and other special needs, such as Down syndrome or cerebral palsy, may also be able to overcome their wetting. If they do not have significant behavior problems and are generally compliant, they are good candidates for what we call the Dry Pants training program. This rigorous approach, which is often facilitated by the medication Ditropan as well as the enuresis alarm, involves establishing a firm schedule of drinking and voiding. Because it is very difficult for parents to carry out the intensive training program at home, the children are generally admitted to the hospital for the first few days of treatment.

the day by age two. It pays to postpone training until your child is clearly ready. If after great patience your child is still not making progress, discuss the issue with your health-care professional.

If your child is due to enter kindergarten and is still not trained during the day, and your health-care professional has ruled out incontinence, we recommend that you use our dryness program as well as a two-tiered reward system: reward your child both for urinating in the toilet and for staying dry between visits to the bathroom (see "Rewarding Daytime Dryness," page 167). If these methods do not work after a couple of months of consistent effort, timed voiding is another option (see "A Voiding Schedule," page 141).

"My son won't get out of bed to pee because he says it's too cold in our house."

During the weeks of treatment, consider raising the thermostat setting to make it easier for your child to leave his bed. Also, leave an extra blanket at the foot of his bed, for him to wrap around himself when he gets up. The bottom line: do whatever you can, within reason, to make your child comfortable.

> *"Well, my son no longer wets the bed, but now he gets up and pees on his bedroom floor. What a mess."*

Consider having him urinate in a bedside commode or urinal temporarily, while you work with him on getting to the toilet at night. Walk with him to the toilet for a few nights, to build his confidence in his ability to move around at night. Also, make sure the path to the bathroom is well lighted. And don't forget to tell him how proud you are of his progress.

> *"My daughter insists that she did not wet the bed, even though the wet sheets are right in front of her. She says that she remembers going to the toilet!"*

Some children dream that they are urinating in the toilet when they are actually lying in bed at the time. Gently and without hostility, explain this phenomenon to your child and help her accept the physical evidence of her wetting.

> *"My seven-year-old girl seems to wet only after she has just finished urinating in the toilet."*

Check to see if she compresses her thighs together forcefully during voiding. If so, the thigh muscles may be redirecting some of the voided urine into the vagina; then, when she stands after finishing, the small amount of urine in the vagina will leak out slowly. The wetness seems to reach the underwear just as the girl is leaving the bathroom.

If your daughter does do this, have her sit farther forward on the toilet seat, with her thighs separated some (this can be hard for obese girls). This position should solve the problem. If it doesn't, consult your doctor.

OPPOSITIONAL BEHAVIOR

Even with their parents' full support and ample offerings of rewards and reinforcements, some children are firmly opposed to getting help for wetting. Such opposition, particularly in children over age eight, usually signals other problems. It is highly unusual for a child to resist treating his wetting problem when it keeps him from participating in social activities. Why would a child be unwilling to help himself? In our experience, such children tend to be angry, depressed, or both.

Angry children consider the treatment program as just one other way in which to defy their parents. If this defiance is part of a pattern of oppositional behavior, having to do with issues besides wetting, we recommend getting your child professional psychological help before attempting treatment of the wetting. If refusal to follow the program seems to be the only symptom of an otherwise well-adjusted child, we recommend talking to the child about his feelings about getting to dry and, then, this very successful first step: having the child take complete responsibility for all of his laundry. Why should you have to do so much additional work if the child is unwilling to accept your help and support to at least try to get dry? Tell your child that if he is willing to work at the program, you will continue to help by doing the laundry. We usually find that after a week or even a few days of doing their own laundry, most children will opt for the treatment program.

"I am Orthodox Jewish. My religion does not favor using electronic devices during the weekly Sabbath."

Because the use of electronic devices on the Sabbath, or Shabbat, is a concern of Jewish laws, there may be uncertainty about the acceptability of using an enuresis alarm during the Shabbat in Jewish homes. Opinions on the practice of Jewish laws and customs may vary regionally, so please consult your local rabbinic authority about use of the alarm. However, according to

Rabbi Asher Lopatin, of Anshe Sholom B'nai Israel Congregation in Chicago, this device and the program can be used on the Sabbath and still be consistent with Orthodox Jewish practice (which normally prohibits completing electric circuits on the Sabbath). Based on the judgment of leading authorities in Jewish law, Rabbi Lopatin finds sufficient mitigating factors and sufficient pressing need to allow the use of the device—especially with children under the age of twelve.

> *"My daughter must just be lazy because when we go on vacations overnight or she spends an overnight at Grandma's, she's dry! At our house she wets!"*

A child's heightened desire to stay dry on vacation or at a relative's house may mitigate the effects of deep sleep and permit her, while asleep, to sense an impending bladder contraction and then stop it. Also, it may not be additional motivation but the fact that while sleeping in a different place, the child does not sleep as deeply. When the child returns to the comfort of her own home, this heightened awareness is gone and wetting may return. In such circumstances, using our program works well: the diaries, the doctor's visit, the diet, wearing the alarm, affixing stickers—all heighten the child's awareness. While the program is *never* intended to be punitive, some children may perceive the treatment as a billboard that shouts, "Pay Attention! The reason you have to measure your pee, wear an alarm, pass up pizza and ice cream for dinner, and take a medication is that you wet the bed. If you can stop the bedwetting, you can return to your routine." This perception may unfairly frighten the child who now sleeps less deeply, so that wetting treatments are more successful.

"My child's night wetting doesn't bother us so much. What we can't fix is that he is dry at school, but wets after returning home."

A child may be apprehensive enough about wetting at school that he focuses on his bladder signals and can stay dry. The school day is also structured, with teachers often providing a bathroom break for students. When he returns to the comfortable setting of his home, he may let his guard down, and wetting happens.

In such cases, it is likely that the bladder capacity is small. Consider a behavior modification program to reward and condition dryness at home using an enuresis alarm, and consult your doctor about the use of oxybutynin (perhaps to use only at home, along with the alarm). If you find that your child's bladder capacity is normal, consider using just the reward program along with the alarm, but no medication. The child should wear the alarm as much as possible at home, to help him be aware of bladder cues when he starts to wet during the day. Keep track of how well the child is doing by using a calendar that divides the day into time periods determined by the frequency with which the child wets.

Some children who wet during the day only at home may do so because of problems in their home life. If the Try for Dry program does not ameliorate your child's wetting, please consult a mental health professional.

"My daughter goes to summer camp next month. How can I get her dry right away?"

First, consult the camp director to find out how they usually respond to such a circumstance. Perhaps they have special advice or instructions for making your child's stay as stress-free as possible.

Also, consider trying DDAVP before she goes to camp as a short-term way of achieving night dryness. The child can continue to take the medication at camp; it is easy to administer and to keep confidential. After camp is over, you can begin the dryness program.

> *"I have a thirteen-year-old girl diagnosed by my family doctor with primary nocturnal enuresis. Her fifteen-year-old brother has the same thing. What type of program should I follow for both children?"*

Because bedwetting has a genetic basis, many parents face the burden of getting more than one child to become dry. Once you have evaluated the children and determined each to have primary enuresis, you can begin using the treatments outlined in Chapters 5 and 6.

However, you need to tailor the program for each child. It may be difficult to give each child an alarm, because it would be going off so frequently during the night that it would be very disruptive for the whole family. Also, it is a good idea to treat the older child first, because if both children are treated simultaneously and the younger sibling happens to get to dry first, the older child may feel frustrated and somewhat humiliated. So work in sequence: first the older child becomes dry, then the younger child.

Not uncommonly, when several children in one family all bedwet and all sleep in the same bedroom, the oldest sibling's participation in the program influences the other siblings to pay more attention to their bladders. When they hear the alarm go off, because the older child wet, they think about their own bladder. So the younger children's wetting may also improve, even though they were not wearing the alarm.

Of course, you are the best judge of your family's situation. In the case of twins, for example, treating bedwetting is particularly challenging. Usually, the less chaotic solution of treating them separately is the best approach.

> *"I think my ten-year-old has a large bladder, not a small one. He hardly ever goes to the bathroom. When he does need to pee, it comes on so suddenly that he tends to get to the toilet too late."*

Some children with enuresis indeed do have a large bladder capacity. They visit the bathroom infrequently, and when they do urinate, they don't completely empty their bladder. Children with such large capacity tend to resist urinating on schedule, because they often do not feel like they have to go.

For such children, we recommend what we call the Drink-Pee-Drink Schedule, which is a daytime regimen of scheduled drinking along with encouragement to void. This schedule is also helpful for children who have a problem with constipation, because it helps keep them well hydrated, so that their stools stay moist. The method also helps children with urine infections, who void too infrequently and drink too little. Explain to your child that you have found a way that might help him stop having accidents. Tell the child that you want him to try to urinate every three to four hours for the next few weeks, so that he can practice feeling the need to pee. Here are the steps to follow:

The Drink-Pee-Drink Schedule

Step 1. Every three to four hours during the day, have your child go to the bathroom. Each time the child enters the bathroom, before he tries to urinate, have him drink four to six ounces of water at the bathroom sink.

Step 2. The child should then try to urinate.

Step 3. After the attempt at voiding, whether successful or not, have the child drink another four to six ounces of water before leaving the bathroom.

Step 4. Repeat this procedure throughout the day, every three to four hours, until the wetting improves.

> *"My sixteen-year-old boy wets at night off and on. He can stay dry for three weeks at a time, but then he'll start wetting several nights a week for months. We've tried a mattress pad alarm, imipramine, and Ditropan. We even had an ultrasound done and his flow rate measured normal."*

In addition to the specific details mentioned above, the child in question had the following characteristics:

- No daytime wetting
- Bladder capacity: thirteen ounces
- Bowel habits: regular stools
- Physical examination: normal
- Diagnosis: enuresis

What makes wetting disappear and then reappear in some children is a mystery. It may relate to unappreciated dietary indiscretions, stool irregularity, or emotional stresses. The first step toward ending the wetting for good is to undertake our dryness program, beginning with Chapter 4. It is likely that the program, if followed consistently, will make a child who wets episodically reliably dry. We have found that when our treatments are followed consistently, wetting relapse episodes happen farther and farther apart, and ultimately remit with continued success.

Should wetting relapse, however, the family should consult an enurologist—that is, a specialist in the field of wetting—or a pediatric urologist about the possibility of incontinence. Keeping a record of daily stresses in your child's life is another option to consider if incontinence is ruled out. (Refer to pages 77–78 of the questionnaire in Chapter 4.)

"A friend of mine told me that hypnosis helped her boy stop wetting. How does that work?"

During hypnotherapy, a child receives suggestions that he retain urine, avoid wetting, and use the toilet when he senses the need to void. What hypnosis accomplishes in the case of enuresis is the means for the child to concentrate on controlling his bladder. For example, you would begin by having your child sit in a relaxed area. Then you would ask your child to imagine that he is in bed and has the urge to urinate. Then you would ask him to imagine getting out of bed, walking to the toilet, and urinating.

Such imagery techniques can be reinforced by talking with your child about wetting, trying to help him understand that he is in control of his bladder. Explain what steps he needs to follow in order to stay dry. Make a drawing together of what it looks like to be lying asleep in bed and feel the need to void, then walking to the toilet, and so on. These techniques help the child to develop better awareness of his bladder's cues of impending wetting.

"My seven-year-old daughter had some problems with bed-wetting while in kindergarten. But now we have more difficulty with day wetting than anything else. She just finished an antibiotic for a urinary tract infection which caused some accidents (both day and night)—but generally, she has a couple of day accidents a week. It's just

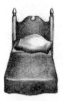

MEMORABLE REAL-LIFE STORIES

Over the years, hundreds of children and their families have come into our lives, some only for a few weeks. Here are a few of our favorite cases:

MOST INVENTIVE

One father of a child we treated had an original idea:

"William's problem is that he sleeps too heavily. We bought one of the enuresis alarms, but it just didn't wake him up. As an engineer, I rigged the alarm so it would not only sound the alarm, but it would also turn on the bedside table lamp. But he still slept through that."

Once William began taking oxybutynin (for small bladder capacity) and following the Happy Bladder Diet, the conventional alarm helped him stop wetting.

MOST ENLIGHTENING

Just when we thought we knew how to take care of wetting, along came "Allen," an eight-year-old boy who had day wetting and night wetting. He wasn't doing that well in school, but that wasn't why we were seeing him.

He just didn't get better with the usual program: alarm, oxybutynin, and diet. His mother was getting frustrated with us, and then

---

enough to put a wet spot on her underwear and most of the time soak her jeans in that area. She is very embarrassed by it.

"I did a voiding diary. . . . The maximum was usually first thing in the morning and never went over four ounces. As you know, this is about half the normal amount for a child her age. There was an ultrasound test, but it was normal.

"She claims she doesn't know when to go and is very adamant about it. I don't think she's lying. She was diagnosed with ADHD, so we thought possibly her 'intense' she started mentioning that his school was on her case about his academic performance. He just wasn't able to focus on his work. So, we suggested an evaluation for attention deficit hyperactivity disorder (ADHD). Perhaps he had trouble focusing on schoolwork as well as on "bladder work."

The evaluation showed the ADHD. After he was treated by his doctor for this, Allen's school and bladder work improved. So did his relations with his siblings at home.

SADDEST

One eight-year-old boy wet every night. His mother got so fed up with her son's wetting that she made him sleep in the bathtub. This did not get him dry.

FUNNIEST

"Dear Dr. Maizels,
   I would like to invite you to my funeral.
   We started the Try for Dry program the night we came home from our office visit with you. I was up about three times at night for the next three nights, then gradually less, and now only a week later we are dry. But I am dead.
   Thank you."

concentration on certain things (such as drawing) might keep her brain too busy to notice. . . .

"We tried Ditropan alone, but it didn't work! Then we tried a voiding schedule, taking her to the bathroom every two hours so she would stop having accidents. This didn't work either. So—as best as I could, I asked her teachers at school to remind her to go to the bathroom, but nothing worked."

Our approach to this problem would start with an evaluation by a wetting specialist—that is, an enurologist—to make sure that the wetting does not result from internal problems of incontinence, such as a condition called vesicoureteral reflux (see Appendix C for more details on this and other conditions related to incontinence). So, while it is good to note that the child's ultrasound test was normal, it could be that a test for reflux would be helpful.

If the reflux test is normal, then there should be no urological problem causing the wetting—that is, incontinence would be effectively ruled out. So for enuresis, even though there was disappointment with the medication in the past, we would suggest using Ditropan again, but *in conjunction with* other treatments suitable for your child's symptoms. (See Chapter 4 to begin the process of evaluating the child's symptoms and then choosing a treatment plan.)

With Ditropan, oftentimes only a small dose is needed, say, one-half teaspoon three times a day. But what makes the child dry is not necessarily the medication, but rather the use of an enuresis alarm during the day. The child can wear the alarm on her hip, like a pager, and let it tell her when it's time to visit the bathroom.

So, although wetting conditions can be complicated by bladder infections, ADHD, or other problems, our approach should be able to match the symptoms with the correct treatments.

Summary

The treatments involving the use of enuresis alarms, medication, bowel programs, and elimination diets usually work. If there are problems getting to dry, however, remember that in order for these treatments to be effective, it is important that you not only follow them as prescribed but also have a complete understanding of *why* they are used:

- The enuresis alarm sounds to wake the *parent;* if the child responds also, then dryness will come faster. Use the alarm consistently.
- A child should take oxybutynin (Ditropan) until the physician says to discontinue it. The medication DDAVP may cause remission of wetting, but if wetting relapses, an alarm treatment should be considered.
- Avoiding an overfull rectum may make it easier for a child to perceive a full bladder. Be sure your child defecates daily.
- In order to isolate and identify any foods or beverages that may be contributing to a child's wetting problems, the elimination diet must be monitored carefully. Be sure that your child does not secretly eat or drink anything he is supposed to be avoiding while on the elimination diet.

In addition, we now realize that in some cases the reason initial treatments do not result in dryness is because of an undiagnosed attention deficit disorder. Once this condition is identified, treatments can be adjusted effectively and successfully, so that now more children are able to get to dry more consistently.

AS A PARENT, or as a caregiver, counselor, babysitter, coach, teacher, or friend, one of the most important things you could ever do for children who wet is to help them get to dry. Achieving dryness not only removes their burden of living with wet clothes and wet sheets but also whatever degree of shame and discouragement the children suffer as a result of their enuresis. It is hard work, and it takes patience and perseverance. But the benefits to the families as a whole are tremendous, and to the individual children who overcome wetting—truly immeasurable.

Appendix A: Glossary

age categories

Infant	Up to two years old
Toddler	Two to four years old
Youth	Five to nine years old
Preteen	Ten to twelve years old
Teen	Thirteen to nineteen years old
Adult	Twenty years or older

behavior therapist   A therapist who is knowledgeable about changing behaviors using behavior modification techniques based on specific learning theories.

bladder   The organ that stores urine until a person is ready to void.

bladder capacity   In this book, we use this term to mean *functional* bladder capacity: the largest amount of urine the bladder can empty at one void (assuming that negligible urine remains inside the bladder after voiding). This is distinct from *anatomic* bladder capacity, which is measured during surgery, while a child is under general anesthesia.

bladder muscles   Two different sets of muscles make up the bladder:

- **bladder sphincter**—The pair of muscles, one of which is situated at the neck of the bladder and the other just beyond the bladder, that retain urine inside the bladder. When the muscles are contracted, the bladder stores its urine.

- **bladder detrusor**—The muscle that lines the bladder. When the muscle contracts, the bladder expels its urine.

constipation   Hard, dry and/or painful stooling. (Compare with **irregular defecation.**)

continent   A child is said to be continent of urine when he can retain urine in the bladder without wetting himself, and when he can discharge the urine into the toilet in a socially acceptable manner at times of his choosing. (Compare with **toilet trained.**)

defecation   The elimination of solid waste; stooling.

desmopressin   A synthetic hormone used to supplement the body's supply of the natural hormone vasopressin, which reduces the volume of urine excreted by the kidneys. The trademark name is DDAVP.

diurnal   A Latin term meaning "by day."

dysuria   Discomfort, commonly experienced as a hot or burning sensation, associated with urination.

encopresis   Fecal soiling of the underpants by a child who is at least four years old.

enema   A liquid, a cathartic, that is instilled into the rectum and colon to stimulate defecation shortly after use.

enuresis   Wetting that is not caused by structural urological or neurological factors in a child who is at least five years old and has never been previously dry for a period of at least six months. Enuresis can be corrected without surgery. (Compare with **incontinence.**) The nature of the wetting can be:

- **primary**—Wetting that occurs in a child who has never had six months of consistent dryness.
- **secondary**—Wetting that occurs in a child who has experienced at least six months of consistent dryness.

- **nocturnal**—Wetting that occurs at night during sleep. (It can also refer to wetting that happens during a daytime nap.)
- **diurnal**—Wetting that occurs during the daytime while the child is awake.

enurologist   A specialist in the treatment of children who wet. Enurologists can be doctors, nurses, psychologists, or paramedical professionals (such as a physical therapist) who have taken extra training.

fecal impaction   A hard, dry plug of stool in the rectum. It must be removed, usually with an enema or occasionally by hand.

giggle wetting   A type of day wetting, most frequently found in girls, that occurs during laughter, giggling, or tickling.

hormone   A substance with biological activity that is produced by an organ and travels via the bloodstream to act upon a distant tissue.

imipramine   A medication used to treat bedwetting. It can have harmful side effects, and so should be used only with careful supervision after it is prescribed by a doctor. The trademark name is Tofranil.

incontinence   Wetting that can be corrected only with surgery because the wetting results from a fault in the urinary tract. (Compare with **enuresis**.)

irregular defecation   Defecation that is not daily.

laxative   An agent that stimulates the bowels to facilitate defecation. Usually taken by mouth, laxatives should be used only after first consulting your doctor. Also called a bowel stimulant. (Compare with **lubricant**.)

lubricant   An agent that softens a hard, dry stool, making it easier to eliminate. Also called a stool softener.

neurogenic bladder   This term refers to any of a variety of conditions of poor bladder function in which the cause relates primarily to a problem of the nerves that serve the bladder. In children, this relates most commonly to spina bifida, in which the nerves to the bladder (and all too often, to other parts of the lower body) are malformed, and so the parts they serve do not function well.

nocturnal   A Latin term meaning "by night."

oxybutynin   A medication that helps a child attain night dryness when used with an enuresis alarm. It is especially useful when the functional bladder capacity is reduced. The trademark name is Ditropan.

pediatric nephrologist   A pediatrician who specializes in medical problems of the kidney and is knowledgeable about problems of enuresis and incontinence.

pediatric psychologist   A psychologist who specializes in working with children who have medical problems as well as behavioral and emotional problems and who has earned a Ph.D. or a Psy.D.

pediatric urologist   A surgeon who evaluates children for incontinence problems related to the urinary tract that could then need to be treated surgically. A pediatric urologist may also be an enurologist so may treat children with enuresis as well as incontinence.

pediatrician   A doctor who specializes in the protection and maintenance of childhood health and the treatment of problems of childhood, including enuresis.

polyuria   The excessive production of urine.

recurrence   Wetting that occurs after *any* interval of dryness.

relapse   Two or more wet episodes (in the daytime or at night) that occur over a two-week interval during the tapering portion of the treatment program or after wetting has remitted (i.e., after fourteen consecutive dry days and nights).

remission Fourteen consecutive dry days and nights within four months after beginning an enuresis treatment plan. There are two further stages of remission:

- **continued success with remission**—No relapse for six months after enuresis treatment is discontinued.
- **complete success with remission**—No relapse for two years after enuresis treatment is discontinued.

scheduled voiding The practice of taking regular trips to the bathroom at predetermined intervals.

sign A finding that a doctor discovers during interaction with a patient (such as discovering reduced functional bladder capacity by examining a voiding diary).

spastic bladder (uninhibited bladder) A bladder that does not show normal "accommodation," the normal expansion to accommodate an increase in the volume of urine *without* an increase in the pressure within the bladder.

suppository A tablet or capsule inserted into the rectum in order to stimulate defecation.

symptom A medical term used to categorize problems patients may complain of (such as bedwetting). (Compare with **sign.**)

toilet trained A child is commonly viewed as toilet trained when the child is continent, or "dry," for at least six months (see **continent**). Unfortunately, it is not uncommon for families to view a child as toilet trained as soon as the child begins wearing underpants instead of diapers, even though the child continues to wet.

urgency The subjective unpleasant sensation of the need to void very soon.

urinary tract infection (UTI)   A condition in which bacteria grow anywhere in the tracts through which urine passes (kidneys, ureter, bladder, urethra) and cause an infection.

urination frequency   The number of times a person urinates on a typical day.

vasopressin   A naturally occurring hormone produced in the pituitary gland that regulates excretion of urine by the kidney. (Compare with **desmopressin.**)

voiding   The act of passing urine. Also known as micturition.

volitional bladder control   The ability to stop a bladder contraction and initiate urination at will.

Appendix B:
The Try for Dry
Song Music

Motivational Verse

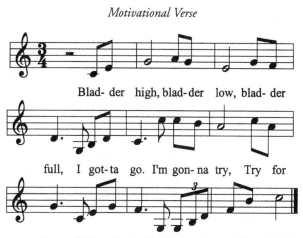

Blad- der high, blad- der low, blad- der

full, I got- ta go. I'm gon- na try, Try for

Dry, & when I do, I'm gon-na be might-y high!

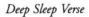

Deep Sleep Verse

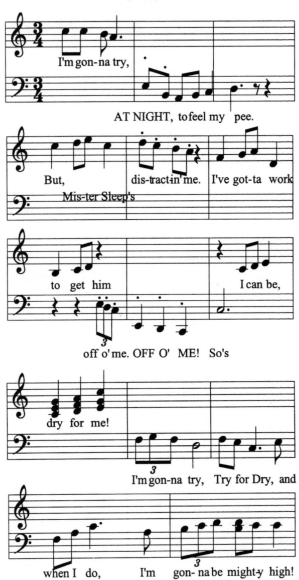

Bladder Size Verse

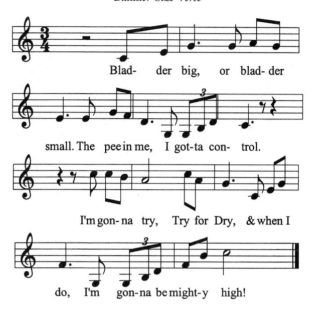

Blad- der big, or blad- der

small. The pee in me, I got-ta con- trol.

I'm gon- na try, Try for Dry, & when I

do, I'm gon-na be might-y high!

Bowel Health Verse

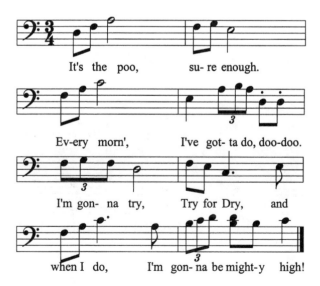

It's the poo, su- re enough.

Ev-ery morn', I've got- ta do, doo-doo.

I'm gon- na try, Try for Dry, and

when I do, I'm gon- na be might-y high!

Diet Verse

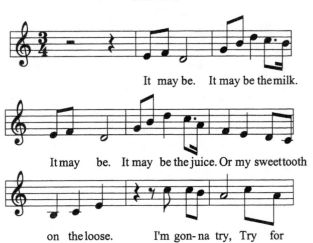

It may be. It may be the milk.

It may be. It may be the juice. Or my sweet tooth

on the loose. I'm gon-na try, Try for

Dry, & when I do, I'm gon-na be might-y high!

Appendix C: Incontinence

About twice a year we encounter children diagnosed with enuresis who have been "waiting to outgrow" their wetting, but it hasn't happened. This is because the correct diagnosis is actually incontinence: the child needs surgery to resolve the wetting. These scenarios are so typical, even though they are infrequent, that it is reasonable to include them here, in case you recognize similarities to your own situation.

When children do not respond to enuresis treatments after three months, we recommend that they be evaluated by a pediatric urologist. After evaluating a child, the pediatric urologist may recommend surgery that will either stop the wetting completely or suggest the child start a new, different dryness program.

The five most common urological conditions that contribute to wetting are

- Posterior urethral valves in boys
- Meatal stenosis in boys
- Ectopic ureters in girls
- Vesicoureteral reflux in boys or in girls
- Spina bifida in boys or in girls

In the following pages, we will briefly describe each of these disorders.

Conditions Specific to Boys

POSTERIOR URETHRAL VALVES

If a boy is wet by day and night and he cannot void with a strong urine stream (for example, he has to stand right up against the toilet in order to have the stream hit the toilet bowl), a condition called *posterior urethral valves* may be the problem. In this condition, a bit of "scar" tissue develops before birth in the region of the developing penis/urethra. This tissue mildly restricts voiding. The bladder commonly becomes "spastic" and small in its functional capacity, and its muscle becomes thick to compensate for the blockage. Many boys with this disorder have to sit when they urinate, because their urine stream is not strong enough to allow them to stand and still have the urine reach the toilet bowl.

Another possible way that posterior urethral valves may cause wetting is that the bladder responds to the blockage of the urethra by "stretching" to *enlarge* the bladder capacity rather than reduce it. A boy's bladder may become so large, and the obstruction so prominent, that he gets tired of waiting for the bladder to empty when he urinates, and consequently he does *not* empty his bladder completely. Wetting follows when the urine leaks because of his still partially full bladder. Doctors suspect this problem when a boy who wets shows a large or larger than predicted normal functional bladder capacity.

This excess tissue can usually be removed with a minor outpatient surgical procedure and without an external skin incision. Once the blockage has been removed, the child then goes on to follow the dryness program.

MEATAL STENOSIS

A small urethral opening at the head of the glans penis may be an example of *meatal stenosis*. If the opening does appear undersized, your child should be checked by a doctor to see if it is indeed too small. The doctor will either observe the force of the urine stream personally or measure the force in a special machine called a flow meter. The condition may cause the boy's urine stream to be thin and forceful—like a stream of water shot from a squirt gun—and therefore showing a "cast distance" much farther than expected.

When the opening at the head of the penis is too small, the bladder has to work harder to empty its urine and, in the process, it thickens. In this state, the bladder muscle becomes irritable. Just as the muscles in your hands and arms may twitch uncontrollably after a long day of clipping shrubbery, your child's bladder may contract uncontrollably while he is asleep.

If your child has meatal stenosis, it is worthwhile for him to follow the dryness program in this book before considering surgical treatment. Children who have a small meatus and are otherwise normal often become dry using this approach. For children who do not respond to the program, however, an outpatient surgical procedure to enlarge the opening (called a meatotomy) may be necessary. After a meatotomy, bedwetting usually subsides either on its own or more commonly in response to a dryness program such as ours. In a few children, bedwetting may actually worsen for a few weeks, until the thickened bladder "softens" back to normal.

A note about girls with a deflected stream: Although deflection of the urine stream is uncommon in girls, we do occasionally see such cases ("It's hard to believe, but when she sits on the toilet to void, her urine stream arcs out of the toilet!"). This misdirection of urine may relate to a web of tissue covering the urethral opening (meatus), as is the case in boys. Or, in some instances, constipation can be so prominent that the stool load in the colon pushes the bladder enough to change the orientation of the urethra, deflecting the voided stream away from the toilet.

Conditions Specific to Girls

ECTOPIC URETERS

Girls who wet by day and night, perhaps even those who are just a little damp, may be showing the effects of an *ectopic ureter*. Occasionally, a little mucus appears on the underpants as well. A girl with this condition typically has a normal bladder capacity, which is a strong tip-off that a problem with incontinence is likely. In such cases, the ureter, which drains the kidney (though usually only the upper portion of the kidney), bypasses the bladder. As a result, the urine made by that portion of the kidney empties not into the bladder but near the vaginal opening. So, in effect, the urine travels directly from the kidney to the underclothes. Only surgery can correct this condition.

Although kidney surgery is certainly complex, it is routine procedure for a pediatric urologist. The surgery usually involves a short stay in the hospital. When the ectopic ureter is identified, it is best to correct it, rather than leave it uncorrected. An uncorrected ectopic ureter will be a continual source of uncontrolled wetting and may also cause a urine infection.

Conditions Found in Both Boys and Girls

VESICOURETERAL REFLUX

Normally, urine travels in only one direction: from the bladder into the toilet bowl. In the condition called *vesicoureteral reflux*, the urine goes in two directions from the bladder: some urine passes as it should into the toilet bowl, but the remainder returns, or refluxes, back to the kidney. Reflux of urine can contribute to urine infections and to wetting problems.

In normal conditions, the kidney delivers urine to the bladder several drops at a time. In cases of reflux, several tablespoons of bladder urine, which have refluxed back up to the kidney, may fall quickly (like a hammer hitting a nail) and hit the nerve-sensitive area of the bladder (called the trigone). It is reasonable to consider that this impact triggers a spastic contraction of the bladder, which, if the child cannot control it, results in wetting.

There is another way in which reflux can contribute to wetting. Normally, when the bladder nears fullness, its internal pressure increases and the child senses the need to void. Once children learn what this perception means, they know that they need to take themselves to the bathroom to urinate. However, in children who have reflux, prior to voiding, the bladder's internal pressure increases normally but then decreases *abnormally* when the urine refluxes back up into the kidney. So the child senses relief from the bladder pressure *without voiding*. These mixed signals seem to confuse the child, and wetting usually follows.

Mild cases of reflux can be treated with medication while children outgrow their problem naturally. Other cases require a surgical procedure to correct the problem. After the reflux has been successfully treated, children usually report that they are able to sense the urge for the bladder release and to control the urge until they reach a toilet.

SPINA BIFIDA OCCULTA

Generally speaking, diseases affecting the central nervous system—the brain and the spinal cord—can impair the functioning of the nerves that serve the bladder muscles. One very unusual condition is spina bifida, in which a spine bone, or vertebra, is incomplete and is evident at birth. The malformation may be so severe that the skin over the lower back is open and the spinal cord may be exposed. Such a severe anomaly is called spinal dysraphism.

A minor form of this anomaly is not overt, but hidden (hence spina bifida *occulta*). In this circumstance, there may be only a slight thickening of a holding ligament of the spinal cord. This ligament may pull too hard on the spinal cord and cause abnormal activity of the nerves to the bladder or weaken the reception of nerves that sense the need to void.

Doctors suspect spina bifida occulta when a child who wets fails to get to dry after following a treatment program and a routine X-ray of the abdomen shows a slight split in a vertebra. Children with spina bifida occulta have been treated successfully with our dryness program. When their wetting does not remit, however, a pediatric urological evaluation should be done. The reason for the persistent wetting may be that the bladder muscle has become overactive because of the faulty nerve connection related to the spina bifida occulta.

This problem can be corrected with surgery. Commonly, the scar band (a thickening of the normal anchor of the spinal cord, the *filum terminale*) acts like a tether at the base of the spinal cord and binds the cord. After the scar band is cut, children usually have more success in getting to dry.

Appendix D: Resources

Suppliers of Enuresis Alarms and Materials

Try for Dry, Ltd.
c/o Reno Lovison Marketing
5250 North Broadway #106
Chicago, IL 60640
(773) 989-1960
E-mail: reno@tryfordry.com
www.tryfordry.com
    Enuresis alarm and materials for hospitals, clinics, and distributors. Try for Dry alarm and materials for individual patients available via the website.

Byram Healthcare
2850 Indian Joe Drive
Broadview, IL 60155
(708) 681-1333
1-800-681-1395
www.byramhealthcare.com
    Distributor of Try for Dry enuresis alarm and materials available by phone.

Nite Train'r Alarm
9735 Southwest Sunshine Court
Suite 100
Beaverton, OR 97005
1-800-544-4240
    Enuresis alarms

PALCO Laboratories
8030 Soquel Avenue, Suite 104
Santa Cruz, CA 95062
(408) 476-3151
1-800-346-4488
   Enuresis alarms

Potty Pager
Ideas for Living
1285 North Cedarbrook
Boulder, CO 80304
(303) 440-8517
1-800-497-6573
   Enuresis alarms

Home Delivery Incontinent Supply Co.
1215 Dielman Industrial Court
Olivette, MO 63132
(314) 997-8771
Fax: (314) 997-0047
   Incontinence products but no enuresis alarms

Harris Communications
VibraLite Watch
(No. GAD-VW)
Voice mail: 1-800-825-6758
Fax: 612-906-1099
   Vibrating alarm wristwatch (You can set multiple alarms to remind your child to visit the toilet and to encourage toileting at appropriate intervals. The alarm vibrates against the wrist, so it is silent and private.)

Odor Eliminators and Incontinence Cleansers

Your local pharmacy, medical supply house, or hospital may stock these products. If they do not, they should be able to help you locate a supplier. (Metro Rehab, listed on page 223, carries most of these.)

Product Name	Manufacturer
Aloe Vesta Cleanser	Convatec/Calgon
Carra Scent Odor Eliminator	Carrington
Citrus II	Beaumont Products
Dignity Odor Eliminator	Dignity
Freshnet Odor Eliminator	Health Point
Hygiene One Cleanser	Bard
Medi-Air Odor Eliminator	Bard
Periwash	Sween/Coloplasty
Triple Core Incontinent Cleanser	Smith & Nephrew
Ultra Fresh Room Deodorizer	Mentor
Ultra Fresh Skin Odor Eliminator	Mentor
Uriwash Skin Cleanser	Smith & Nephrew

Bed Protectors

Just as with odor eliminators and incontinence cleansers, ask your local pharmacy, medical supply house, or hospital for these products.

For the Bed
Dignity Plus Sheet/Linen Protector
Priva Self Quilt Reusable Bed Pads
Serenity Waterproof Mattress & Pillow Covers
Tranquility Slimline Pouch Sheet Care Pads

For the Child to Wear
Depends Disposable Underpads
Prevent Plus Boys, Girls
Rejoice Extra Care
Salk Deluxe
GoodNites (www.goodnites.com)

For Additional Help

Try for Dry Program in Pediatric Enurology
Max Maizels, M.D., Diane Rosenbaum, Ph.D.,
  Barbara Keating, R.N., M.S.
Division of Urology
The Children's Memorial Hospital
2300 Children's Plaza, Box 24
Chicago, IL 60614
(773) 880-4428, 8:30 to 4:30 Central Time
Fax: (773) 880-3339
http://www.tryfordry.com

National Association for Continence
P.O. Box 8310
Spartanburg, SC 29305
(864) 579-7900
1-800-BLADDER

National Enuresis Society
7777 Forest Lane C727
Dallas, TX 75230
1-800-637-8080
http://www.peds.umn.edu/Centers/NES/

Spina Bifida Association of America
4590 MacArthur Boulevard, NW, Suite 250
Washington, DC 20007
(202) 944-3285
1-800-621-3141

Continence Restored
407 Strawberry Hill Lane
Stamford, CT 06902
(914) 285-1470

National Kidney Foundation Enuresis Hotline
1-800-622-9010
1-888-WAKEDRY

The Simon Foundation for Continence
P.O. Box 815
Wilmette, IL 60091
(847) 864-3913
1-800-23-SIMON (1-800-237-4660)

Evanston Continence Center
1000 Central Street, Suite 730
Evanston, IL 60201
(847) 570-2750

Publications of E.R.I.C.
Enuresis Resource and Information Center
65 St. Michael's Hill
Bristol BS2 8DZ
UNITED KINGDOM
Telephone: 027 226 4920

The Continence Foundation of U.K.
2 Doughty Street
London WC1N 2PH
ENGLAND
Telephone: 071 404 6875

The Continence Foundation of Australia
Level 1, 59 Victoria Parade
Collongwood, Victoria 3066
AUSTRALIA
Telephone: 03 9419 2163

Aventis Pasteur Inc.
DDAVP
www.drynights.com

References

Clark, Donna. "Gentle Remedies for Bedwetting." *Mothering*, Winter 1994, 46.

Glicklich, Lucille Barash. "An Historical Account of Enuresis." *Pediatrics* 8 (1951): 859–76.

Golbin, Alexander Z. *The World of Children's Sleep.* Salt Lake City: Michaelis Medical Publishing Corporation, 1995.

Hall, Janet. *How You Can Be Boss of the Bladder.* Melbourne, Australia: The Competent Care Consultancy, 1989.

Hogg, Ronald J., and Douglas A. Husmann. "The Role of Family History in Predicting Response to Desmopressin in Nocturnal Enuresis." *Journal of Urology* 150 (1993): 444–45.

Mack, Alison. *Dry All Night.* Boston: Little, Brown and Company, 1989.

Maizels, Max, Kevin Gandhi, Barbara Keating, and Diane Rosenbaum. "Diagnosis and Treatment for Children Who Cannot Control Urination." *Current Problems in Pediatrics* 23 (1993): 402–50.

Scharf, Martin. *Waking Up Dry: How to End Bedwetting Forever.* Cincinnati: Writer's Digest Books, 1986.

Schmitt, B. D. "Nocturnal Enuresis: Finding the Treatment That Fits the Child." *Contemporary Pediatrics* (1990): 70–97.

Tietjen, D. N., and Douglas A. Husmann. "Nocturnal Enuresis: A Guide to Evaluation and Treatment." *Mayo Clinic Proceedings* 71 (9): 857–62, 1996.

Index

About the Authors

Max Maizels received his medical degree from UCLA Medical School in 1973 and completed urology training at Chicago's Northwestern University Medical School in 1980. He is a professor of urology and has been in academic and clinical practice at the Children's Memorial Hospital in Chicago since 1980. He is also the director of the Institute for the Unborn Baby in Chicago. His primary clinical interests include enuresis and urological problems of the fetus.

Diane Rosenbaum received her doctorate in clinical psychology from Washington University in St. Louis. She has been a clinical psychologist at Chicago's Children's Memorial Hospital since 1982, providing psychological services to children and their families. She specializes in pediatric psychology and is the psychologist for the Try for Dry program. She also has a private practice in the greater Chicago area.

Barbara Keating received her nursing degree from DePaul University in Chicago, and her master's degree in science and nursing from Northwestern University. She has been caring for children at Children's Memorial Hospital for eighteen years. She coordinates pediatric urological care, particularly for enuretic children and for children with myelomeningocele.

Notes